Smart Women
Strong Bones

Revised Edition

Ronda Gates, M.S., C.L.C.
Beverly Whipple, Ph.D., R.N., F.A.A.N.

Smart Women

Strong Bones

Revised Edition

Ronda Gates, M.S., C.L.C.
Beverly Whipple, Ph.D., R.N., F.A.A.N.

LIFESTYLES Four Heart Press
Lake Oswego, OR

ALSO BY RONDA GATES
The Lowfat Lifestyle
Nutrition Nuggets/Changes: The Rest of the Story
Smart Eating: Choosing Wisely, Living Lean
with Covert Bailey
The Scale Companion
with Frank Katch, Ph.D. and Victor Katch, Ph.D.
Beauty, It's More than Skin Deep
LIFESTYLES PLANNER weight management software

ALSO BY BEVERLY WHIPPLE
The G Spot and Other Recent Discoveries about Human Sexuality
with Alice Kahn Ladas, Ed.D., and John D. Perry, Ph.D.
Safe Encounters: How Women Can Say Yes to Pleasure and
No to Unsafe Sex with Gina Ogden, Ph.D.

Publisher's Cataloging-in-Publication
(Provided by Quality Books, Inc.)

Gates, Ronda.
Smart women, strong bones / by Ronda Gates, Beverly Whipple. — 2nd ed.
p. cm.
LCCN: 00108287
ISBN: 1-878319-02-7
1. Osteoporosis in women. 2. Osteoporosis in women—Prevention I. Whipple,
Beverly. II Title.

RC931.073G38 2000   616.7'16
                                                         QBI00-901467

Cover Design and Illustrations by Dale Lamson, Lamson Design, Cincinnati, OH
Text design by Sheryl Mehary
Published by LIFESTYLES 4Heart Press, a division of
LIFESTYLES by Ronda Gates

Introduction

Several years ago I'd never given any thought to osteoporosis. I wasn't even sure what it meant. I figured it was something that happened to women much, much older than I was. Then, because I have a small frame and am Caucasian, my doctor suggested I have a DEXA scan to determine if I had osteoporosis.

There was no one more surprised than I was to learn that *I did have osteoporosis.* I had exercised most of my life and I followed a good diet. I didn't smoke. I certainly didn't have a dowager's hump and I didn't want one. I especially didn't want to give up my active lifestyle or healthy sex life. It's hard to enjoy both of these without strong bones. I also wanted to be able to play with my grandchildren.

If you attend a Speaking of Women's Health event this year, you will learn that lost bone can be replaced with an active lifestyle, good diet, calcium supplementation, and a powerful, proven medication called Actonel® (risedronate sodium tablets). Actonel® is a prescription medication for postmenopausal women at risk for osteoporosis.

I was put on Actonel® to help my bones become healthier and more fracture-resistant. After taking Actonel® for a year another DEXA scan revealed there was marked improvement in my bone density. Of course, Actonel® is not right for everyone, and your results may be different. It is important to talk to your doctor about your risk for fracture and whether Actonel® is right for you.

I hope you will take the hour you will need to read this important little book. The information inside and Actonel® are certainly making a difference for me.

Florence Henderson
Honorary Chair
National Speaking of Women's Health Foundation

You should not take Actonel® if you have low blood calcium, severe kidney disease, or cannot sit or stand for 30 minutes. Stop taking Actonel® and tell your doctor if you experience difficult or painful swallowing, chest pain, or severe or continuing heartburn as these may be signs of serious upper digestive problems. Side effects are generally mild or moderate and may include stomach pain or upset, or constipation. Follow dosing instructions carefully.

Contents

Appendix

Acknowledgments

Every published book is the creation of more than its authors. In this case, friends took what we thought was a stellar project and returned it to us covered with red marks, suggestions for revised phrasing, and questions. "I don't know what this means," or "You already said this," or "A whole chapter could be developed on this topic." We discovered our egos can survive constructive criticism, sort through feedback, and accept suggestions that clarified everything we were trying to say. Each draft (and there were many) was better.

These are the people who made *Smart Women, Strong Bones* possible:

In Ronda's office:
Janice Hoffman, for her willingness to edit and compile resources.

Tami Jewell, for coordinating logistics and adding her eagle eye to the proofing process.

Caleb Gates, for the perspective of a man reading a book written for women.

In Beverly's office:
Jim Whipple, for manning the computer, when it wouldn't perform as expected.

Sue Whipple Forcier, **RN**, **MS**, for the younger woman's perspective.

Pat Bessey, for the middle-aged woman's perspective.

Lois Ann Kastl and **Vivian Heiler**, for helping us remember what is important to women as they get older.

English teachers and editors are our worst enemies and best friends. Thanks to **Sophie Ravis**, who was willing to read and edit from the perspective of a woman and grammarian. Her husband, **Howard Ravis**, a former editor, added to this perspective.

Dr. Robert Lindsay, our highly respected physician, friend, and the former President of the National Osteoporosis Foundation who generously read and edited our text and contributed the foreword.

Dr. Lana Holstein, author of *Magnificent Sex* and Women's Health Director at Canyon Ranch Health Resort and **Dr. Marisa Weiss**, author of *Living Beyond Breast Cancer* and president of www.breastcancer.org, our friends and Speaking of Women's Health colleagues whose perspectives, as women and physicians, assured our content included practical advice for our readers.

Dianne Dunkelman, the awesome and energetic visionary, backbone, and founder of Speaking of Women's Health Foundation. Dianne supported us through every page and provided feedback based on her experience with thousands of women whose lives she has touched. With her help, the idea for this book, forged during a passionate discussion about women's health issues, became a reality.

Foreword
by Robert Lindsay, M.D.

Osteoporosis is gradually being recognized as a major health problem for women. However, it is not a new problem. The changes in body configuration that occur with osteoporosis can be found in writings as old as the 2nd century B. C. when Hippocrates, the father of medicine, described the rounded back that is the hallmark of spinal fractures caused by osteoporosis.

What is new about osteoporosis is that more women are living long enough to be at risk for the disease. As they age, they are certain to experience the estrogen deficiency that follows menopause (or the surgical removal of the ovaries). That deficiency precipitates the bone loss that leads to osteoporosis, the dowager's hump, and easily fractured bones that are signatures of advanced disease.

Baby boomers, just entering menopause, have precipitated heightened interest in this disease. They want, indeed demand, to age with good health. Happily we can give them good news. Osteoporosis can now be prevented. Women who have osteoporosis can be diagnosed and treated before any fractures occur. That is why this book is so timely. Readers will learn good health habits that can prevent the disease, and how it can be diagnosed and treated in the early stages, before devastating effects, including the signature dowager's hump and other broken bones, temper an active life.

Beverly and Ronda are masters at providing practical applications for the information they deliver, including how to start an exercise program, options for supplementation, and the background that enables women to ask the right questions of their health-care providers. They also describe, in easy-to-understand, everyday language, the currently available bone-density tests that can measure just how much bone tissue is present, how the tests are interpreted, and the variety of treatment options currently available, as well as a preview of what the future holds in this important arena.

For those of you most at risk for the disease, or those who already are stricken with osteoporosis, this book will be an invaluable resource, helping you to navigate the process of deciding which of the available therapies is the most appropriate for you. This choice can be difficult. Should it be hormone replacement therapy, a tissue selective estrogen, or a bone specific drug such as a bisphosphonate or calcitonin? What role can calcium or other supplements play? Since treatments are taken for a long time, perhaps in some instances lifelong, it is important that the patient be comfortable with the choice that is being made. The decision process requires dialog between the patient and her health-care provider. This timely and very useful book empowers women. It is a thoroughly readable and enjoyable volume that goes a long way toward assisting in that difficult process of becoming a well informed and active participant. This book supports a longer healthy life.

Prologue

Our Stories

Once upon a time, the standard of health care for women was designed by and based on what we knew about men. Women were banned from drug trials for 20 years. Until 1993, all medical research was oriented to men. Scientists learned how men's bodies metabolized food, responded to exercise, and got sick and well, then extrapolated that information and applied it to women. Most physicians, pharmacists, and researchers were men. They told us how to take care of ourselves and, in most cases, we yielded to their authority. If women wanted to help people be well, we were relegated to roles as nursing assistants, research assistants, technologists, and health educators.

Happily the face of women's health has changed. We have many more options than our mothers or grandmothers. Women must be included in all drug studies. When we seek medical care, we meet female physicians, nurse practitioners, and pharmacists. We've discovered we have options so we ask questions, seek alternatives, and discuss these options with friends and families. Thanks to programs like "Speaking of Women's Health," we expand our educational horizons and realize we have choices. Many of these new choices contribute to our ability to take control of our destiny and have a longer, more fulfilling, and healthier life.

Sadly, not everyone has received the message. Compare these three scenarios. Which of these women will you be?

Ruth

In 1993 Ruth was a vibrant 80-year-old woman in the middle of her second adulthood. She flourished in her role as a highly visible community leader whose efforts to promote health education earned well-deserved accolades and a humanitarian award from the University of North Carolina Board of Directors.

One morning, just after her 80th birthday, Ruth awakened with an all too familiar tightness in her chest. She used the bronchodilator prescribed for allergies and bronchospasms, took her thyroid medication and vitamins, ate breakfast, and "went to work." Later in the day, she was paralyzed by a bronchospasm that literally "rattled her bones" when she coughed. When she finally caught her breath, she felt exhausted. Her back hurt. She decided the "coughing spell" had given her a muscle spasm but she didn't let it stop her. Her stiffness increased and the discomfort in her back became more severe. By the next morning the slightest movement precipitated excruciating pain. A friend drove her to the hospital where x-rays revealed that she had five spontaneous spinal fractures. Ruth was diagnosed with osteoporosis.

Seven years later, this 87-year-old woman is seven inches shorter and has a dowager's hump. She uses a walker to prevent a fall. The last time she got in and out of a car it precipitated three more painful spinal fractures, so she no longer leaves her home. Her mobility there is limited to walking from her bed, where she spends most of her time, to her kitchen table where, because her appetite has diminished, she eats only a few bites of the few foods that satisfy her. She is in constant pain, which she alleviates with codeine and muscle relaxants that have, over time, diminished her mental capabilities. She is scared. Most of her friends died long ago, so she is lonely. And she is angry. All these emotions are projected on the caretakers and family who have attempted to give her the support she needs. Yell and complain to friends and family long enough, and the friends stop calling.

Jean

Jean is Ruth's 52-year-old daughter. She's learned her lesson well. After the wake-up call delivered by her mother's diagnosis in 1993, she decided to adopt an osteoporosis-preventing lifestyle. She joined and used a health club. She agreed to hormone replacement therapy despite concerns about its long-term use. She began taking a calcium supplement. So you can imagine her surprise when she received the results of her first DEXA scan this year. It showed she has osteopenia, a loss of bone. In Jean's case it's noticeable in her hip, pelvis, and shoulder. Although this news devastated her, her doctor wasn't so distressed. After cheering Jean's efforts for the past seven years, she told her, "Your bone loss would probably have been worse if you'd been more sedentary these last seven years. Keep up the good work." She added the good news that because there are new drug treatments to prevent bone loss, women no longer need to face the agony and pain caused by deteriorating bones. Jean shared her doctor's excitement when she learned that a new class of drugs formerly used to treat Paget's disease (another bone disease) were now approved to treat osteopenia and osteoporosis. "Tell your women friends not to despair if they have been diagnosed with osteoporosis. They should contact their doctors so they can learn how these miracle drugs that actually improve bone density and significantly decrease the risk of fracture can become part of a comprehensive treatment model." Jean agreed she would spread the word.

Ann

Ann is Jean's 28-year-old daughter. She's been physically active all her life. She doesn't smoke or diet excessively. Her alcohol consumption is limited to an occasional glass of wine with dinner. She's heeded media information about good nutrition, takes a supplement of calcium and vitamin D and, since her grandmother's diagnosis, follows the guidelines for prevention of osteoporosis. Her DEXA scan shows her bones are typical (strong) for a woman her age. Since she is predisposed to osteoporosis, she plans to continue her active lifestyle. Unless there are unforeseen circumstances (a chronic illness, for example), she can expect to live into her second or third adulthood with the choices available to healthy, active, osteoporosis-free women.

Osteoporosis

Osteoporosis is a condition that was not widespread until medical and technological advances for diagnosis and treatment of disease increased a woman's life span. As they lived longer, more and more women developed osteoporosis. Here are alarming statistics every woman should know:
- Today, 45 percent of postmenopausal caucasian women have osteoporosis.
- One woman in 10 over age 65 has a collapsed vertebrae.
- By age 80, forty percent of all white women in the United States will sustain a hip fracture if they fall.

The good news is that women don't have to wait until they experience a fracture to discover that their bones are becoming more fragile. There are assessments that can predict risk and get women treated early. Best of all, a majority of the risk factors that predispose women to osteoporosis are lifestyle factors. Empowered with the knowledge and resources you will gain here, each of us can temper or prevent a disease state that leads to painful elderly years.

In order to make wise choices women need accurate, useful, easy-to-understand information. Thanks to organizations like the Speaking of Women's Health Foundation, women attending day long conferences nationwide are learning they have choices that can impact their lives and the lives of their family. We hope this book will contribute to this effort.

Ronda and Beverly

Introduction to Revised Edition

What an experience this book has been! More than 30,000 copies of the first edition of *Smart Women, Strong Bones* were published and delivered to individuals and audiences nationwide. Interest in the book precipitated a revised edition, published early in 2001, which sold an additional 40,000 copies. Now we are in our third edition with new information and the prospect of distribution to thousands more readers, thanks to the endorsement and support of Florence Henderson. This warm, delightful woman has heightened the awareness that osteoporosis is a serious disease. Indeed, osteoporosis has been highlighted in all media venues triggering action by women who want to assure they reach the end of their life without a disease related fracture. They are asking, and in many instances, demanding their doctor order a bone density scan. They are also asking health insurance carriers to pay for these scans. Physicians are seeking the most up-to-date, authoritative medical information and guidelines on the disease. Medical research is advancing rapidly as funds dedicated to the prevention and treatment of this life-threatening disease have increased by more than 10 million dollars.

Not all the news was good. New research shattered the myth that osteoporosis is an old lady's disease. A study in Arkansas revealed that in a group of over 100 women ages 18-30 more than fifteen percent already have lower than normal bone mass. Several had already crossed the threshold to a diagnosis of osteoporosis. In depth examination of the data revealed the cohort of women with disease were low weight women who did not exercise or strength train but dieted to remain thin. Another study revealed teens who consume lots of soft drinks have a lower bone mass. We learned that more mothers are giving their young sons and daughters tooth decaying juice instead of bone building milk for snacks.

In the last edition you met three real women struggling with a variety of osteoporosis-related issues. Since then Ruth has continued to deteriorate. She cancelled the twice weekly visits by a physical therapist designed to retain muscle strength, increase balance, and maintain flexibility because the sessions were too painful. This set the stage for more fractures, a smaller lung capacity, and advancement of diseases that exacerbate without activity including the congestive heart disease and accompanying shortness of breath that is now so frightening she rarely leaves her bed.

Jean remained committed to the exercise program, hormone replacement, and supplement therapy she hoped would prevent her from becoming "a little old lady" like her mother. She added strength training, flexibility, balance and agility training to her routine and discovered aging didn't mean slowing down. Jean preached the "get a bone scan" message to her peers and when she learned a close friend was taking the new miracle bisphosphonates on an irregular basis, gave her a copy of our book and reminded her that taking her medicine was as important as brushing her teeth.

Jean's daughter, Ann, also continued her active lifestyle. She "came out of the closet" and admitted that for a short period of time when she was in college she struggled with an eating disorder. Now she's an advisor to a support group for young women who are trying to reverse body image issues.

Every week we have excitedly exchanged information we've received that updates or highlights osteoporosis issues. In this edition we've distilled them and sprinkled them throughout the text to give new and former readers a fresh look at a preventable disease. Though choosing which feedback to highlight was difficult, we're sharing some of the quotes we received from grateful readers. You will also find reports on the results of research studies published since our first edition, and an updated appendix. Overall, this is, we believe, the most "up to speed" book on the strategies you can use to prevent and treat osteoporosis and, forever be a Smart Woman with Strong Bones.

Please continue to write and tell us about your experiences. We care.

Ronda and Beverly

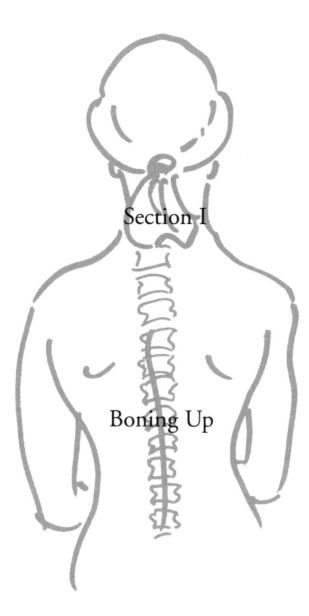

Section I

Boning Up

"I was surprised to discover osteoporosis is a woman-killer."

Deidre, Age 44

Chapter One

The Other Life-
Threatening Disease

"I learned a lot about bones that I didn't know."

Diane, Age 76

What is Osteoporosis?

Most women know aging brings an increased risk of declining health and multiple diseases. We have watched women friends, acquaintances, and parents age and die. We are used to hearing about deaths from heart disease, stroke, or cancer. But few of us are aware of another killer that steals more women's lives than breast cancer. It is osteoporosis.

Osteoporosis used to be considered a natural part of life for an aging woman. That is no longer true. Today this common human bone disease is diagnosed in the old and the young. Nevertheless, it is middle-aged women who are newly aware of osteoporosis as an important health issue. It is well described by its name: Osteo = bones and Porosis = porous. Osteoporosis literally means "porous bones."

Important Facts You Need to Know

- Osteoporosis is characterized by low bone mass and an increase in the risk of fracture.
- Osteoporosis affects more than 25 million women in the U. S.
- Osteoporosis will cause a broken bone in one out of every two white women over age 50. There is also significant risk, although it is lower, for non-white women and for men.
- Osteoporosis is the cause of more than 1.5 million spine, hip, and wrist fractures in the United States each year. These fractures affect one out of every six women.
- One in five women who sustains a hip fracture dies within one year of complications precipitated by the bed rest required for recovery.
- In the United States, costs for fractures from osteoporosis are in excess of $15 billion a year.
- If women in their 30s and 40s don't take preventative action, it is estimated that by the year 2020, costs for osteoporosis-related fractures will be $60 billion annually.

Women Take Notice!
Unfortunately, most women don't find out they have osteoporosis until they fracture a bone, notice they have lost height, or develop curvature of the spine. In fact, one of the first symptoms may be back pain. That is why osteoporosis, like high blood pressure or heart disease, is called a "silent" disease. It can progress without outward signs while, internally, potentially devastating consequences loom on the health horizon. Osteoporosis is a risk factor for fracture just as high blood pressure is a risk factor for stroke. Osteoporosis is like high blood pressure in another way. It can be prevented and treated with a combination of lifestyle, diet, and therapeutic approaches.

"Do Women Really Live Longer or Do They Just Take Longer to Die?"

One of the consequences of living a long time includes a decline in the body systems that function so optimally when we are young. One of these is the ability to maintain bone density. Both men and women lose some bone mass as they age. People with osteoporosis have lost an excessive amount of bone. The bone that is left is so porous, brittle, fragile, and weakened that it can snap under stresses that would not break a normal bone.

Bone Loss

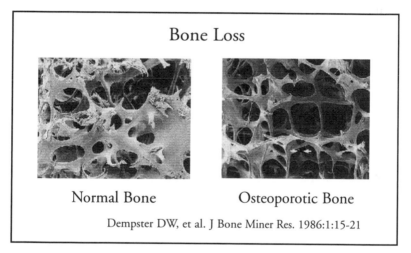

Normal Bone   Osteoporotic Bone

Dempster DW, et al. J Bone Miner Res. 1986:1:15-21

If the bone that breaks is a hip bone, return to a previous level of activity is rare. One in five women die from complications like pneumonia and blood clots that are precipitated by the required bed rest. Statistics reveal that more than half of the women who suffer a hip fracture need help with the activities of daily living. Nearly one-third of them are forced to move into long-term care facilities. Fear, anxiety, and depression are common when women live with this disease. What woman would look forward to this lifestyle?

When You Don't Have Osteoporosis

You don't have to be diagnosed with osteoporosis to be affected by the disease. Nearly three quarters of the friends and relatives who provide care for osteoporosis patients are women, with 85 percent of these women over age 45. Described as "the sandwich generation" because they care for children *and* parents, these essential and overlooked caregivers have a critical role that will be compromised if they, too, fall victim to osteoporosis. That's the bad news. There is also good news. The dismal future described above may be tempered soon. Scientists have provided us with new knowledge of how bone mass increases, peaks, and declines. We can examine risk factors and do tests that measure the density of our bones. Researchers have eagerly embraced this information to explore new options for the prevention and treatment of osteoporosis. These exciting new drugs will change the face of this disease and, if you do your part, enhance the quality of your life.

> Thanks to new drug therapy, women no longer have to suffer the constant pain, limited lifestyle, and complications that come with osteoporosis.

What You Need To Know:

By following the guidelines offered in this book, you can take charge of your life and your health. You can help prevent osteoporosis in yourself, in your daughters, and, as new drugs that reverse this disease emerge, help your mothers—even if they already have the disease. Read on!

Chapter Two

Why Women Are Different

"Thanks for making menopause easy to understand."
Angie, Age 45

Of course, women are different. It's obvious, and it's about more than physical appearance. They think and communicate differently. Whole books have been written about the different speaking styles of men and women. Women are different on the inside too. Their different reproductive organs produce different hormones, which have different functions. All these differences play a big role in the diseases we might develop as we age. That's why researchers, doctors, and women coming to health conferences talk about "gender-specific biology."

Although both men and women get osteoporosis, the surging and receding hormones that accompany a woman's menstrual cycle contribute to the heightened risk, earlier onset, and overall prognosis of osteoporosis. We can't talk about osteoporosis in men or women without talking about how the human body functions.

Sex hormones are important for acquiring and maintaining bone mass in both men and women. Testosterone is the primary hormone for men, while estrogen is the primary hormone for women, although both men and women have testosterone and estrogen. These hormones escalate at puberty and subside as we age. However, estrogen declines faster and more abruptly in women than testosterone does in men. For women, the most apparent changes happen at the start of menstruation, at puberty, and when menopause begins in middle age.

How Menstruation Works

The human body is remarkable. Most of the time it works in a complex feedback system, much the same way a thermostat responds to the temperature of your home. In a woman's reproductive, or sexual system, her two reproductive organs, the ovaries, regulate the thermostat. Each ovary contains structures called follicles, which hold egg cells. A woman is born with about 500,000 egg cells. By puberty, about 75,000 are left. Only about 400-500 of these egg cells fully mature. The rest degenerate. The female body also produces many hormones. Four of these, estrogen, progesterone, the follicle-stimulating hormone (FSH), and the luteinizing hormone (LH), are the active hormones of a woman's menstrual cycle. Just after menstruation begins, when estrogen and progesterone levels are low, one of the action oriented brain centers, the hypothalamus, begins to work. It stimulates the pituitary gland, which releases FSH and LH. The follicle, now stimulated by FSH and LH, produces the sex hormones estrogen and progesterone. This causes the lining of the uterus to thicken, becoming a potential source of nourishment for the development of one or more fertilized eggs. If male sperm does not fertilize the egg, the lining of the uterus breaks down, menstruation occurs, and the cycle begins again. Like the thermostat, low levels of estrogen and progesterone begin the action of FSH and LH. High levels of estrogen and progesterone turn off that action.

Perimenopause and Menopause

The "change" of life, when powerful estrogen levels decline significantly, and the cyclical pattern of menstruation gradually stops, is a marker for women in many ways. Until recently, we didn't know much about perimenopause, and didn't talk about menopause. We didn't know much because at the turn of the 20th-century, not many women lived past menopause. We didn't discuss it because it was an "embarrassing" subject and a life passage dreaded by many women. Menopause signaled aging, and in the U. S. we remain phobic about getting older. Even in our more enlightened times, precipitated by the thousands of baby boomers beginning to move into this phase of life, there are still many myths and misconceptions about menopause. In a survey asking women what was the worst thing about menopause, most said, "Not knowing what to expect is frightening."

Medically, the word menopause means the permanent end of menstruation. It is derived from the Greek words for "month" (mensis) and "cessation" (pausis). Menopause is a normal stage of a woman's life triggered by a decrease in estrogen levels. This transition is a process that can take as few as five or more than 10 years. Even women as young as 35-years-old experience perfectly normal physical and emotional symptoms of menopause. Perimenopause is the start of the transition, when women have fluctuating hormone levels and irregular ovulation.

The hormonal changes that take place during perimenopause and menopause are not unlike those that take place during puberty and pregnancy. There are pleasures but there may also be emotional swings. Smart women think of menopause as a period in their life when they are likely to be "hormonally challenged."

> Typically, this transition in a woman's life is divided into three phases:
>
> **Perimenopause:** the start of the transition-that time immediately prior to naturally occurring menopause when the changes indicating the approach of menopause begin
>
> **Menopause:** the completion of the ovarian transition, marked by the last menstrual period (menopause is considered complete when a woman has not had a menstrual period for one year)
>
> **Postmenopausal zest:** the time women tap into a new vitality

Just as each woman experiences puberty and pregnancy differently, each goes through perimenopause and menopause in her own way. We have different levels of hormones circulating in our body, different diet patterns, exercise patterns, and life experiences. All affect our physiology. That is why the menopause experience can range from virtually no symptoms, except the cessation of menstrual periods, to long-lasting symptoms, which severely interfere with day-to-day living. Most of these reactions are prompted by three factors:
1. The level of circulating hormones.
2. The intensity of hormonal changes.
3. A woman's sensitivity to her hormonal changes.

Ten to fifteen percent of women breeze through this time with no discomfort, while another ten to fifteen percent experience severe symptoms. The majority of women (seventy-five to eighty percent) have one or more peri-menopausal symptoms that are inconvenient but manageable. Even though we call these 'symptoms,' it is important to remember menopause is not a disease but a normal phase of life.

Symptoms of perimenopause and menopause that some women experience include:

Insomnia	Night awakenings
Hot flashes	Breast tenderness
Headaches	Heart palpitations
Joint pains	Frequent urination
Fatigue	Irregular periods
Irritability	Vaginal dryness
Moodiness	Lack of sexual desire
Memory loss	Pain with intercourse
Night sweats	Mental sluggishness
Unusual skin sensitivities	

It is unlikely every woman will experience all these symptoms. That's the good news. The bad news is none of them are a welcome intrusion to daily life.

Smart women overcome the experiences that accompany menopause with a positive attitude. Hot flashes become "power surges." Vaginal dryness becomes an "Astroglide" opportunity, and memory loss becomes a "senior moment." A change in attitude can change everything.

It's All About Hormones

In a woman's mid-thirties, the ovaries begin to decline in hormone production. This process accelerates as a woman reaches her mid-to-late forties when hormone levels fluctuate even more, causing irregular cycles and heavy bleeding. Estrogen is still produced in small amounts by the ovaries. Another form of estrogen, estrone, is produced in fat cells.

Interestingly, heavy women whose weight predisposes them to other diseases experience less symptoms of perimenopause and menopause.

More fat cells = more estrone = less symptoms of menopause.

As a woman approaches menopause her levels of estrogen and progesterone begin to drop, her supply of eggs dwindles, and the follicles lose their ability to respond to the FSH and LH stimulation. FSH and LH levels increase in an effort to make the ovaries produce more estrogen and progesterone.

Lower levels of estrogen and/or progesterone can result in periods of moodiness and depression. One reason is that the ovarian hormones interact with endorphins, biochemical substances in the brain that act like "internal morphine." Endorphins can block feelings of pain and give women a sense of well-being.

When women have both ovaries surgically removed, they experience an abrupt menopause. This surgery, known as a bilateral ovariectomy (or bilateral oophorectomy), usually occurs at an earlier age than naturally-occurring menopause and these women may be hit harder by the symptoms of menopause than women who move to this stage as a natural process of life. Additionally, women who have chemotherapy, or radiation to their pelvic area, can also experience premature ovarian failure. And there are 10 percent of women who fall outside the expected norms for menopause and stop menstruating before their 40th birthday.

Menopause Signals Bone Loss

As menopause begins and estrogen levels start to decline, women are more susceptible to bone loss. Estrogen deficiency is clearly associated with osteoporosis. The advent of menopause accelerates age-related loss of bone mass, with a greater loss in trabecular bone than cortical bone. (You will learn more about the various types of bone in the next chapter.) By contrast, prolonged estrogen exposure, which happens when puberty is early, menopause is late, a women uses birth control pills, or has had a baby, helps increase and sustain bone. That doesn't mean women should wait until menopause to start taking care of their bones. We teach our children there are delayed rewards for depositing money in a bank, studying for a test, or training for a competition. They should also be taught their health will profit if they begin, now, to practice behaviors that will decrease their risk for osteoporosis in their future. That includes lessons in how to achieve peak bone mass with regular exercise and a nutritious diet that includes lots of calcium-rich foods.

The percentage of women in the United States who experience natural menopause, by age:

AGE	PERCENTILE
38	10
44	30
49	50
54	90
58	100

What You Need to Know:

Menopause is not the end of a woman's life; it is the beginning of a new phase of her life. Knowledge of what to expect can empower a woman to make the most of it. We are now in an era of health care when physician's instructions are not blindly accepted. Patients ask questions. Women today do have a say in their physical and emotional well being. See our appendix for suggested questions for your doctor.

Chapter Three

Bones — A Life and Death Story

"Thanks for teaching us how bones work."

Nancy, Age 22

Two-year-old, Isabella, one of Ronda's younger friends, was in a traumatic accident last year. She was standing near some boards propped against a garage wall, watching her brothers play ping pong. The ball got away from the boys and rolled behind the boards. During the boys' enthusiastic pursuit to retrieve the ball, the boards were knocked over on Isabella, resulting in a spiral fracture of her thigh. After surgery to reset the fractured bone, both of her legs were molded into a plaster cast, rendering her immobile from the waist down for six weeks. It saddened me to see this formerly active child lying on her back in a red wagon, pulled by her mother or father from room to room, or lying immobile on the floor, watching videos.

Two weeks later, Isabella was pulling herself anywhere she wanted to go by the sheer brute force of her arms. She was no longer on pain killing medications so she slept and woke at normal hours. Although it was a difficult time for Isabella and her family, they were coping.

Last week, only three months after the accident, Ronda was stunned when she visited the family again. Isabella was running all over the place. There were no ill effects from her injury. When asked how she was doing, her mother shrugged her shoulders, shook her head, and replied with amazement, "Great!"

Two years ago Ronda, at age 58, had a wicked, ankle-twisting fall. She was certain the ankle was broken. It wasn't. Her doctor told her he believed her active lifestyle created strong bones that withstood the violent twisting motion and resulted in only a severe sprain. Despite a commitment to her rehabilitation, and what her doctor called "a remarkably quick recovery," it was many months before the injury was only a vague memory.

These two incidents are a vivid comparison of how our body responds to injury at different ages. We exist in an incredibly efficient machine that constantly builds, breaks down, and repairs tissue throughout life. Unfortunately, as we age, the speed at which that process occurs slows down considerably.

Our bones are no exception to this process of change. When we are young, and growing, new bone is forming all the time. In adolescence, when children experience accelerated growth spurts, we often hear them complain that their bones ache—signs the bones are working overtime to lay down new tissue. But while bone is forming, it is also breaking down. Until we reach our mid-twenties or early thirties, the bone building exceeds the breakdown process. In our thirties, buildup and breakdown is about equal. Soon breakdown exceeds formation and we begin to "lose" bone. This constant building and breaking down occurs from the smallest bone in our ear to the largest bone in our thigh.

Even the biggest bones are not hard through and through because there are two parts to bone. The biggest, about eighty percent of our skeletal system, is the hard outer bone that protects and supports internal organs and resists the stresses of every day life. This compact outer bone is called **cortical** bone. It is what you see when you look at a skeleton. About eighty percent of cortical bone is "calcified," which gives it a dense quality.

There is also an "inner" part of bone called **trabecular** bone. It is only about twenty percent calcified. It is more spongy, porous, and flexible than cortical bone. Like a sponge, these qualities give it more surface area. Trabecular bone provides the "give" that prevents hard bone from breaking until it is subjected to strong compression or extreme mechanical stress.

When we are infants, none of our bones are hard. Instead, they are mostly composed of a rubbery substance called cartilage that, with the exception of the lengthening ends (called "epiphyseal growth plates"), harden by a process called ossification. Only that tiny bone in our ear, which remains soft throughout life, escapes the hardening processs.

There Are Two Parts to Bone:

Cortical bone is the strong, compact outer bone. Bones in the arms and legs are mostly **Cortical** bone.

Trabecular bone is the spongy, porous, more flexible bone. The ribs, jaw, and the spine are mostly **Trabecular** bone.

The lower part of the wrist is about 2/3 **Trabecular** and 1/3 **Cortical** bone.

Ossification takes place because bones contain busy cells called osteoblasts. These cells are like masons putting bricks together to build a house. They build (or rebuild) bones and store the calcium and phosphorous (from our diet) that makes bones hard. Unless the osteoblasts are diseased, nothing stops these busy cells from the constant bone-building process.

Osteoblasts are stimulated by the female hormone estrogen, the male hormone testosterone, and the growth hormone from the pituitary gland. All act as messengers to tell the osteoblasts to work hard. These hormones have another supportive tool, calcium. When your body is fed enough calcium, the osteoblasts continue to work hard, encouraging an ongoing bone-building cycle

Like a house that is constantly changing, there is also a demolition and recovery team in the bones. It is composed of other hard working cells called osteoclasts. Osteoclasts release acids and enzymes, which chew strong bones apart. They deposit calcium, phosphorous, and protein by-products into the blood stream for use in other parts of your body. As they work, they leave tiny channels behind to be rebuilt by the osteoblasts.

If the osteoblasts work overtime, bones become deformed. If the osteoclasts work overtime, bones become weak.

Remember these words:

OSTEOBLASTS are BONE BUILDERS.

OSTEOCLASTS are BONE BREAKERS.

Until adolescence is over, because the ends of the bones are soft, they increase in length. As we move from adolescence into our mid-twenties, the work of the osteoblasts exceeds that of the osteoclasts. Bones increase in mass, or density, as these bone-building cells build thicker walls. This bone building process reaches its peak in the trabecular inner bone in our mid-twenties. Our outer cortical bone continues to build, peaking several years later. These early years are the critical times when we have an opportunity to adopt habits that optimize bone health. After this, there is a period of time when bone formation and resorption are about equal. By our late 30s or early 40s, when male and female hormone levels start to decline (long before menopause), resorption starts to accelerate and there is a loss of bone, mostly in the long bones of the arm and leg. The speed of loss is based on genetics and lifestyle factors including exercise, smoking, and diet. Once a woman begins menopause, her decreased ovarian function reduces the production of estrogen and her bone loss accelerates considerably–about six times more rapidly than a man of the same age. If she does nothing to prevent this loss, her bone–especially the porous trabecular bone–can recede in density to the low levels of adolescence.

The Role of Calcium

Throughout life, your body, which considers calcium a pivotal mineral in countless every day functions, constantly monitors its supply. If there is not a lot of calcium in your system because you:
1.   avoid calcium-rich dairy products
2.   lead a sedentary lifestyle
3.   smoke
4.   drink lots of alcohol
5.   take corticosteroids or other bone-robbing drugs
your bones get a message that the systems requiring calcium to function optimally must make some adjustments. A kind of telephone tag begins. Low calcium levels trigger the parathy-

roid gland to secrete a hormone that signals the bone-building osteoblasts to quit storing calcium. They, in turn, tell the osteoclasts to break down bone to release more calcium into the bloodstream. Low calcium levels also signal the kidneys to hold on to any calcium about to be eliminated in urine. Additionally, the kidneys, which have been storing the vitamin D you acquire through sunlight, supplements, or fortified milk, convert those vitamin D stores into an active form, calcitrol. Calcitrol makes the body more efficient at absorbing calcium, making it easier for the parathyroid to get a hormone based message to the bone.

CALCIUM keeps nerve impulses flowing

CALCIUM allows muscles to contract properly

CALCIUM is integral to blood clotting

CALCIUM helps regulate hormone balance

CALCIUM initiates metabolic pathways

What You Need to Know:

If you could look at live bone, you wouldn't see any activity. You might think it is stable and not very active. Nothing could be farther from the truth. Bone is dynamic and alive, actively attempting to maintain the delicate balance between osteoblasts that build bone and osteoclasts that break it down. The bone building process, taking place in both the hard cortical bone and soft trabecular bone tissue, is at its peak early in life. It is this bone mass attained early in life that may be the most important determinant of life-long skeletal health. A balanced, high calcium diet and regular exercise contribute significantly to the efficiency of this process, which peaks about age 30. Dietary calcium also plays a role in many physiological functions of the body. When you don't get enough calcium in your diet, the body "steals" calcium from your bones to maintain proper blood calcium levels for this other "more important" work.

Osteoporosis is not always the result of bone loss. **Your early (and current) eating and exercise behaviors, combined with genetics, hormone changes, and other lifestyle factors, determine whether peak bone mass will be maintained.** If it is optimized when bone is forming then maintained with healthy lifestyle habits you will not get osteoporosis. If bone mass declines until the cortical bone is thin and the once uniform, honeycomb-shaped trabecular bone becomes irregular and enlarged, you will be left with frail bone that is easily fractured. You will be diagnosed with osteoporosis. It's a life and death choice you can control. Read on to learn why and how.

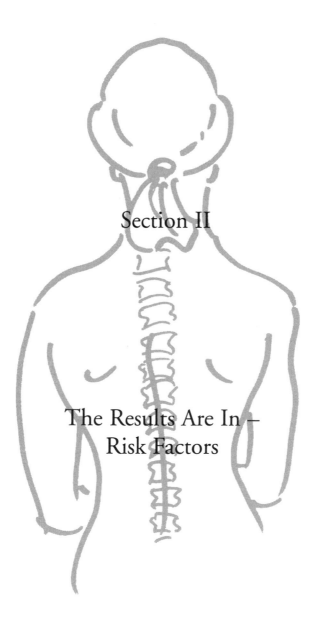

Section II

The Results Are In –
Risk Factors

"I thought everyone who got old would eventually get a humped back. Now I know better."

Julie, aged 44

Chapter Four

Your Genes — More
Than a Pair of Pants

*"My grandmother has a dowager's hump, but I won't
let it happen to me."*

Jacqueline, Age 31

Perhaps your mother or grandmother is like Ruth, whom you met at the beginning of this book. If so, you may be looking into your own future. As you look into your crystal ball, do you see brittle bones or a dowager's hump? Do you see yourself afraid to go out because you may fall and break your hip? Before you wrap yourself in foam, let's take a realistic look at your unalterable osteoporosis risk factors.

Why do some women develop osteoporosis but others do not?

Many of the reasons we get osteoporosis can be traced to our ancestors. When it comes to genes, the best thing you can have going for you is an osteoporosis-free family history. We also know other uncontrollable factors, including gender, race, small body frame, or a predisposition to poor calcium absorption, can increase your risk for the disease. There is interesting research evolving that suggests a genetic predisposition to alcoholism, one of the risk factors for osteoporosis. Regardless, this remains a lifestyle issue because, despite family tendencies, we have choices regarding lifestyle behaviors.

These Encourage Bone Density
- Parents with strong bones
- Physical activity at every age
- A nutritionally adequate, calcium-rich diet

These Can Foster Loss Of Bone
- Menopause
- Age-related bone changes
- Decline in physical activity or no physical activity at a young age
- Impaired absorption of calcium
- Adverse effects of other medical conditions
- Adverse effects of drugs

Risk Factors Explored

Gender: As you learned in Chapter 2, being a woman puts you at greater risk for developing osteoporosis than being a man. Women have less bone than men to begin with. They have smaller muscles to move those bones and they lose bone mass more rapidly than men. There are lots of terrific advantages to being a woman. Your risk for osteoporosis is not one of them.

Race/Ethnicity: Caucasian (white) and Asian women are the most prone to osteoporosis. Studies reveal that fewer

African-American, Native-American, and Hispanic women experience the disease. They are not, however, without risk, and should take the same preventative measures as their more predisposed sisters.

Genetics: Studies of twins and comparisons of mothers and daughters indicate approximately 60 to 80 percent of the factors contributing to bone density are genetically determined. If your mother had a fracture, your risk for fracture is doubled.

Look at your older relatives for signs you are vulnerable to this disease. Red flags include any loss of height with aging, curvature of the spine (commonly known as "dowager's hump"), fractures in later years, and/or chronic back pain. In Chapter 1 you learned back pain may be one of the first symptoms of osteoporosis.

Genetics play a strong role in the development of many diseases. Osteoporosis is no exception.

The brothers and sisters of people with osteoporosis are six times more likely to suffer from low bone mineral density than the general population.

Bone structure and body weight: Thin, petite women, described by physiologists as ectomorphs, are more vulnerable to osteoporosis than mesomorphic, bulkier body types. Taller and heavier women have bigger and denser bones and a lower risk for osteoporosis. Heavier women naturally produce more estrogen from their fat cells. That gives them more protection against osteoporosis than thin women, but this advantage over their thinner sisters is slight.

Women with eating disorders, especially anorexia, often have a fragile body structure and low body weight that gives them an appearance that can be misinterpreted as a genetic predisposition to be small. Scientists are studying the brain chemistry and certain brain centers of women with this aberrant lifestyle to determine if there is a genetic and/or biochemical link that predisposes them to these behaviors. Regardless of the outcome, eating disorders, crash dieting, over-exercising, and the too lean frame they can precipitate, are risk factors for osteoporosis.

NOTE: Calorie restriction combined with the estrogen deficiency that makes women stop menstruating is a serious threat to current and long term health.

What Is a Woman to Do?

If you are like us, daughters of women with osteo-porosis, you may wonder, "Am I doomed to get osteoporosis?"

The answer is, "No." You have the power to overcome a genetic, race, or gender-based predisposition for osteoporosis by making the best of the risk factors you can control. While you practice healthy, osteoporosis-preventing-behaviors, we will keep our ear to the ground for you. There are many genes currently being studied in an attempt to identify a specific gene for osteoporosis. It would be wonderful if we could be tested at an early age to discover if we are at risk for osteo-porosis—much as women whose mothers died of breast cancer can be tested today. Women who are adopted or whose mother died at an early age could gain information not currently available to them. So far, the resulting data for an osteoporosis gene are unclear. Meantime, read on to learn about other risk factors, testing, and treatment for osteoporosis and the prevention strategies that will make you a smart woman with strong bones.

What You Need to Know:

Although it's impossible to change your gender, race, frame size, or your family history of osteoporosis, you are not doomed to repeat the past. There are alterable risk factors for osteoporosis that can change your predisposition to this disease. If you make them a priority now, your future can be a healthy one.

Chapter Five

Risk Factors: Self-Defeating Behaviors

"Everyone should know how bad dieting is for the bones."

Julie, Age 35

Diet

If you could see a biochemistry chart, you might be surprised to learn how essential vitamins and minerals are to life. They play a vital role in every cell. They help move oxygen through your blood, build cells for your eyes, help muscles contract, and increase the density of your bones.

Suddenly it becomes easier to understand why it is important for children to have an adequate diet. When children are deprived of the vitamins and minerals they need to grow, they have a delayed puberty. That creates risk factors for many diseases later in life, including osteoporosis. Although all nutrients are important, the need for calcium, to provide early prevention against osteoporosis, is sufficient reason for us to tell children, "Drink your milk."

There are many resources that explore the role between diet and osteoporosis in depth. The American Dairy Council and its state organizations do a terrific job of teaching kids of all ages about the benefits of dairy products. You can also consult your library or the Internet for additional resources.

As we move through puberty to adulthood, up to two percent of our total body weight is the calcium in our bones. That calcium comes from our diet. That is why it is important, for adults, as well as children, to make use of the milk food group foods. Despite this knowledge, many "experts" tell us we don't need to drink milk after puberty. We hear, "Animals don't drink milk after they are weaned, so why should humans?" That argument is insane. Female animals don't have to worry about menopause. They are physically active and don't live long enough to get osteoporosis. WOMEN DO! THINK ABOUT IT.

If you don't drink milk, you need to be more aggressive about getting your calcium from other dairy products (and other calcium rich or calcium fortified foods). If you choose a milk-free-diet because you are "lactose intolerant," there are over-the-counter products at your drugstore that can relieve the "gas" caused by an inability to break down milk sugars. Bottom line: **If milk and dairy products aren't a part of your diet, it is essential you work with a dietitian to be sure you get the nutrients you are missing when you eliminate this important food group from your diet. You could pay with your life.**

High Protein Diets

As this book goes to press, there is a resurgence in the promotion of high protein diets for weight loss. Although there are hundreds of studies proving weight management is about balancing calories in and calories out, we continue to hear from hucksters who have their pocketbook, not your health, as their motivation for perpetuating these crash diet myths.

Most Americans already eat much more protein than their bodies need. When they do, their body must metabolize the excess. Proteins are nothing more than a grouping of amino acids. Osteoclasts remove bone more easily in an acid environment. You can see how a high protein diet that puts lots of amino acids in the blood could set the bone depleting osteoclastic activity, described in Chapter 3, in motion. This cycle can be a setup for an increased risk of osteoporosis, especially if it is combined with a low intake of calcium rich foods.

Women who buy into the high protein diet weight loss strategy should be aware it can be dangerous to their bones.

Interestingly, some studies show that vegetarians have a lower incidence of osteoporosis than meat eaters. Although the jury is still out and other factors could be involved (do vegetarians, as a group, exercise more or smoke less than meat eaters?), this relationship is of interest to those of us eager to learn everything we can about preventing this tragic disease.

Eating Disorders

Some women who struggle with body image or control issues adopt behaviors that give them an illusory sense of control but seriously compromise their mental and physical health—including their gynecological and bone health.

Bulimia is a "binge and purge" eating disorder. It is characterized by eating excessive amounts of food in a short period of time. This gorging typically continues until it is interrupted by the severe discomfort of feeling full. This awareness triggers an intense fear of weight gain that precipitates self-induced vomiting, fasting, abuse of laxatives, use of diet pills or diuretics, and excessive exercise.

Bulimia is a serious health problem that most frequently affects women in late adolescence or young adulthood. Its cause is complex and, since people with bulimia are usually normal weight, it often goes unrecognized.

When a woman continues a cycle of binges and purges, her body becomes depleted of water and potassium. When purging methods include the use of laxatives, bone density also decreases. As this disease progresses, it can be a signal to the body that reproductive health is not good. Menstruation becomes irregular or ceases. This change in estrogen level precipitates osteoporosis.

Exercise Bulimia is a less well-known form of bulimia characterized by a food intake-exercise relationship designed to maintain weight. People who suffer from exercise bulimia are terrified of getting fat. The potential enjoyment of each meal is tempered by obsessive thoughts and accompanied by a plan for the exercise that must occur to prevent any fat storage. There is an appearance of good health and physical fitness, but the exercise has nothing to do with health benefits. Sadly, the fitness community often supports this disease. Exercise instructors think little of encouraging people to exercise to "burn off those calories" eaten at an earlier meal or to create the calorie deficit that gives them permission to eat more at the next meal. Most women who have issues about their body image or weight practice some form of exercise bulimia, which has erroneously been described as a positive addiction. Although exercise bulimia doesn't directly precipitate osteoporosis, it is often one of the steps that leads to the bone-robbing diseases of bulimia and anorexia. It is also an acceptable "recovery" route for former bulimics.

Anorexia Nervosa is a more serious eating disorder believed to be rooted in issues of control. There is also an unrealistic fear of becoming fat that has the hallmark of an unrealistic self-perception of body size. Anorexics have a preoccupation with food, calories, and food preparation. They encourage others to eat while they, themselves, engage in severe self-restriction of food intake that leads to drastic weight loss. When practiced for a lengthy period of time, there is a loss of calorie burning muscle, which gives them an emaciated look. Anorexia is most common in adolescent girls and young women, who perhaps, for emotional reasons, practice this behavior in an effort to maintain the appearance of small children.

Women with anorexia have irregular or non-existent menstrual cycles. They also have significantly reduced bone mass and, therefore, an increased risk of bone fractures later in life. One study that treated recovering anorexics with a proper diet, calcium supplementation, exercise, and estrogen therapy resulted in weight gain but no improvement in bone mass.

Sadly, as this book is written, there are many high-profile actresses and models pursuing this excessively thin look to counter the effects of television and photographic cameras that make us look heavier than we are. The fashion world also plays a role. Emaciated, at-risk-for-osteoporosis looking models who grace magazine covers and appear in advertisements, provide pressure that encourages young women to be dangerously thin. Additionally, the professional dance community promotes an image encouraged by some choreographers who like their dancers to be skinny and bird-like. These women, on pointed toe, often experience fractures of their fragile feet and legs.

Despite recent books and articles that reveal abnormally thin women will pay a psychological and physiological price in later years as their activity decreases and their bodies experience the changes that come with menopause, the belief that women cannot be too thin drives too many toward dangerous health consequences–including fragile bones.

Excessive pursuit of thinness affects bone health.

Exercise

Ask anyone you meet, "Is exercise important to good health?" Unless they've been in a cave, their answer would be, "Yes," even if they don't exercise. Study after study reaffirms the benefits of exercise. Even anthropologists who unearth bones thousands of years old discover that one forearm bone of our ancestors was enlarged, leading to the conclusion that slinging spears, boomerangs, bolas, and stones exercised the muscles and strengthened the bones in the dominant arm. Research labs confirm what we already know. People who exercise have denser and stronger bones. Pay attention! Positive changes take place in all sedentary people who begin to exercise, regardless of their age.

If lack of exercise is such a significant predictor of whether we will or will not develop osteoporosis, why do so many women procrastinate?

An active lifestyle in the early years of life encourages bone density.

An active lifestyle in the middle and late years of life retains or rebuilds bone density.

Perhaps too many of us remember exercise built on the mantra, "No pain, no gain." That may have been the operating rule when exercise was taught by sergeants with clipboards and whistles, but it is not true. Bone building exercise requires effort. It shouldn't be painful.

We also have "busy" lives, filled with commitments to others. "I don't have time," is the typical excuse. Consider this. If you wanted to lose a dress size for your high school reunion, wouldn't you make time to exercise? If you knew a big deposit in your bank account would be the reward for an investment in exercise, wouldn't you adjust your priorities?

We remind people, "If you don't exercise now, you may not be able to do the activities you can enjoy later in life." Too many respond, "That's OK. I deserve to sit around later." Then later comes and, with it, the pain of fragile bones and a dowager's hump that make sitting around painful.

Smart exercisers set measurable goals and build in their own rewards. They find creative ways to stay motivated. For many, a commitment to friends to share exercise time works best. For others, time set aside for "working out" can be a relaxing, introspective, and invigorating time alone. Remember there is truth to the mantra: "Use it or lose it."

There is one population group that does not benefit from exercise. Women who exercise so much that they stop menstruating (called amenorrhea) are women who have very low levels of estrogen. It is as though the body says, "You have so depleted your resources, I refuse to support a new life." Studies show these women have a significantly lower mineral density in the spine along the lower back. If these women stop over-exercising, then are treated with hormone replacement therapy, they will maintain the bone they have, but will not replace the lost bone.

Doctors agree. If exercise could be packaged in a pill, it would be the most prescribed drug in the world today. Take our advice. Climb steps, lift weights, use a treadmill, take a long walk in the fresh air. Your bones will love it.

Caffeine

If caffeine were discovered today, it would be banned from our diet because of its extraordinary addictive properties. It sends us racing to the bathroom. It keeps us awake. Nevertheless, we are willing to spend several dollars a day to get our physical and physiological fix. No substance has been the subject of more urgent health bulletins – all mutually contradictory – than caffeine.

Researchers continue to attempt to clarify conflicting research about a link between caffeine and cancer, caffeine and heart disease, and caffeine and osteoporosis. One study calculated that calcium loss, from the use of as little as 40 mg of caffeine a day, added up to a ten to fifteen percent bone loss per decade. Another study refuted the first when the subjects chosen didn't smoke or use alcohol. However, since exercisers rarely smoke and often choose to avoid alcohol, that could have accounted for the difference.

> If you prefer caffeinated coffee or tea, consider adding extra milk to offset the calcium draining effects of caffeine.

It takes only 300 mg of caffeine (about two cups of coffee) to cause your body to excrete 15 mg of calcium and other important minerals. This amount may seem insignificant when we consider total calcium is about 2 percent of our body weight. But since little things can add up, it seems wise for people at risk for osteoporosis, especially older women, to go the non-caffeine route as often as possible.

CAFFEINE — IS IT WORTH THE LIFT?

Source	Milligrams of caffeine
Colas (12 oz.)	
Jolt Cola	100 mg
Sugar-Free Mr. Pibb	58.8 mg
Mountain Dew	54 mg
Tab	46.8 mg
Coca-Cola	45.6 mg
Diet Coke	45.6 mg
Pepsi Cola	38.4 mg
Coffee And Tea	
6 oz. Fresh Drip Coffee	115-175 mg
6 oz. Brewed Coffee	90-140 mg
6 oz. Instant Coffee	66-100 mg
6 oz. Decaffeinated Coffee	2-4 mg
6 oz. Hot Tea	30-100 mg
1.5 oz. Shot Espresso	100 mg
12 oz. Iced Tea	70 mg
Chocolate	
1 oz. of chocolate bar	15 mg
1 oz. Baking chocolate, unsweetened, Bakers	25 mg
Pain Killers (per pill)	
Excedrin	65 mg
Anacin	32 mg
Cold Medicine (check the label)	
Other Over-The-Counter Pills (per pill)	
Vivarin	100 mg
NoDoz	100 mg

Smoking

Back when it was cool to smoke, we saw slim, wrinkle-faced, dowager-humped women sitting around with cigarettes hanging out of their mouths. They knew about the addictive properties of nicotine but had little awareness their habit was destroying their bones.

Cigarettes deactivate your production of estrogen. (Remember, estrogen encourages osteoblasts to build bones.) Women who smoke tend to go through menopause earlier than women who don't smoke, adding extra years of low estrogen production and, subsequently, more bone loss.

If you used to smoke and are now smoke-free, good for you. If you haven't given up nicotine—yet, try one of the excellent smoke cessation programs available. End your use of this life-threatening drug. The resource section in the Appendix of this book has a few suggestions.

Alcohol

If you like a glass or two of wine with dinner you probably cheered when research revealed a moderate consumption of alcohol can have a positive effect on heart health. This news is a good example of the saying, "Statistics are like bikinis; they reveal only part of the truth." What the highly publicized media reports forgot to add is that a little alcohol may be helpful but a lot of alcohol interferes with calcium absorption, increasing the risk of osteoporosis. A review of the health charts of alcoholics reveals it's true. They have a much higher incidence of osteoporosis than the non-drinking population. Alcoholics tend to drink their calories. They tend to have a low-in-vitamin-and-mineral diet. The axiom "falling down drunk" can have severe repercussions for women whose bones get fragile because they overuse or become addicted to this potent drug. Enjoy a glass or two of wine or beer, but remember, moderation in all things is the best course of action.

When You Have No Choice — Chemotherapy

Ronda's friend, Nancy, recently was diagnosed and successfully treated for breast cancer. Nancy is five feet tall and has a small frame that would predispose her to osteoporosis anyhow. Her active lifestyle, which includes teaching fitness classes, cycling, hiking, and in winter, skiing kept her bones strong-until she had chemotherapy. After her course of treatment was over Nancy celebrated a full return to her active lifestyle. Then, one day, while skiing, she took a fall that would not break an average person's bones but broke Nancy's leg in several places. Her recovery included months in a wheel-chair, then physical therapy, and a slow re-introduction to her lifestyle. Happily, Nancy is fully recovered but her warning to all women who have breast cancer to have a bone scan before and after chemotherapy is supported by researchers. Women who survive breast cancer are at double risk; they experience menopause early as a result of their treatment, which leads to increased bone loss. Additionally, they are not candidates for hormone replacement therapy, which prevents osteoporosis. The close to the story is a good one. Nancy is now on a bisphosphonate, rebuilding bone and doing well.

What You Need to Know:

Most people who want to change self-defeating behaviors (including yo-yo dieting, failing to exercise, too much coffee, smoking, or alcohol) say, "I know what I need to do, but I just can't seem to do it." The compulsive quality of all these behaviors has repercussions in all areas of life. In short, if you want to be active and bone healthy in your elder years, you must take responsibility for your errant ways today, not tomorrow. Every moment counts.

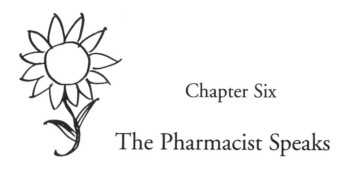

Chapter Six

The Pharmacist Speaks

"I had no idea a prescription could be harmful to my bones."

Margaret, Age 72

Do you use drugs?

Your first reaction to the question may be a resolute "No!" because this question often refers to drugs that are self-administered and abused. In fact, those of us who use a wide variety of pills and potions every day think nothing of it. Whether it is an over-the-counter purchase to alleviate a minor symptom, a prescription from your physician to prevent or treat a disease, or the use of food, herbs, or other supplements, drug use has become a part of modern life.

When taken as directed, prescription and non-prescription drugs, supplements, and foods can effectively treat many symptoms and illnesses. That is the good news. There is accompanying bad news. Most medication works on more than one site or system of the body. For every positive action derived from the use of a drug there is almost always an accompanying message to the brain and body that elicits an unrecognized or unwanted response.

Ruth, described in our introduction, took thyroid medication after she received a diagnosis of hypothyroidism (an under-active thyroid) in her mid-thirties. The prescription stabilized her symptoms. However, the blood tests available at that time to determine an appropriate dose could only tell the doctor if she was receiving too little thyroid. Recently developed tests to measure thyroid are much more sophisticated. They include a test called a TSH, which measures the amount of thyroid stimulating hormone in the blood. A high TSH means thyroid production is low. If TSH is low, the patient is getting too much thyroid medication. By the time Ruth's TSH revealed her current dose could be lowered, she already had more than twenty years of excessive therapy in her system. That extra, unnecessary medication contributed to her fragile bones and set the stage for the compression fractures of her spine at age eighty.

There are many medicines, in addition to thyroid, which have undesirable effects on the health of our bones. Because, most of the time, you need these medicines to treat other diseases, it is important to understand which drugs affect bones so you can be more diligent about taking the necessary steps to prevent osteoporosis if you use them.

Bone Busting Drugs

Thyroid Medication

The glands of the body are very tiny, but they pack a powerful punch. The thyroid may be the most powerful of all. This two-lobed gland is about the size of a thumb. It sits on the front of the lower part of the neck. The thyroid gland produces three hormones important for the functions we call metabolism. The amount of hormone produced by the thyroid is regulated by the thyroid stimulating hormone (TSH), which is located in another powerful gland, the pituitary. If your thyroid is over stimulated, the diagnosis is hyperthyroidism — a syndrome marked by a fast metabolism that can make you feel very energetic, give you a slight hand tremor, and cause you to lose weight. If your thyroid is under stimulated, your diagnosis is hypothyroidism — a syndrome that can make you feel very sluggish and cause weight gain.

For a long time, thyroid medication was extracted from the thyroid gland of a cow and it was difficult to regulate the dose. So, like Ruth, many people received too much medication and lost bone, experiencing all the symptoms of osteoporosis, including fractures. Now most doctors use one of the many synthetic thyroid extracts that delivers a powerful punch in a small dose. Doctors can precisely measure the correct dose for each patient by testing blood TSH levels. If the result is normal, the patient is receiving the correct dose and the doctor doesn't worry about drug-induced osteoporosis. If the TSH is low, the patient is getting too much thyroid replacement. The dose can be adjusted to prevent bone loss.

If you feel tired and sluggish and know you are perimenopausal or menopausal, be sure to report these symptoms to your doctor. Your blood will be drawn and a TSH test ordered to discover whether the cause of your symptoms is or is not hypothyroidism. If it is, you will receive a prescription for medication you should take daily. A follow up blood test will be scheduled to make sure your thyroid is now at optimum function but not compromising the health of your bones.

Corticosteroids
(sometimes called adrenocorticosteroids or steroids)

The term corticosteroids describes many powerful drugs that mimic the action of the adrenal glands. These two small glands, about the size of the end section of your thumb, sit on top of your kidneys. They produce cortisone-like chemicals, including sex hormones, hormones that convert starchy foods into the storage form of sugar, and hormones that maintain fluid balance and reduce inflammation. When you have an adrenal deficiency (Addison's Disease) or a disease state, like asthma, lupus, or arthritis, the long–term use of corticosteroids will reduce swelling, pain, redness, and heat. Corticosteroids are also used to treat certain skin diseases and some cancers.

Oral use of corticosteroids for a week or two, injection of the drug into a joint or excessive scar tissue, or use of topical preparations will produce the desired effect of the drug with no residual side effects. However, multiple short treatments or long term use of these remarkable medications by people who have normal adrenal function, can decrease the action of bone forming osteoblasts and the absorption of calcium that can last for a long time after the drug has been discontinued. The urine of people who use corticosteroids shows an increased amount of calcium, meaning there is an ongoing increase in bone loss. In other words, corticosteroids destroy the bone-building and enhance the bone-breakdown process. This produces a potentially severe bone loss that makes the spine and ribs susceptible to fractures with the slightest trauma.

If your doctor prescribes cortisone, hydrocortisone, or one of their modified forms, like prednisone (5mg or more for more than 2 months), you need to be sure you are practicing as many bone-loss prevention strategies as possible. (See Chapters 12-15.)

NOTE: Never stop taking steroids just because you read that they can harm your bones. Instead, talk with your doctor about the appropriateness of the dose and the duration of treatment you are getting.

The more common steroid prescription drugs are:

Aristicort®	Cortisone®	Medrol®
Celestone®	Decadron®	Prednisolone
Cortef®	Deltasone®	Prednisone

Diuretics

Diuretics are drugs that increase urine volume. They treat high blood pressure and congestive heart failure by decreasing blood volume and, subsequently, the workload of the heart. Like most drugs, there are several classes of diuretics. Only one of them, the loop diuretics (which get their name because they work in an area of the kidney called Henle's Loop) cause the kidney to excrete excess calcium. If you take Lasix®, Aldactone®, Dyazide®, Bumes®, Diamox®, or Edecrin®, you need to drink additional water, add extra calcium to your diet and, with your doctor's permission, participate in an ongoing exercise program.

NOTE: Loop diuretics are so good at removing calcium from the body that they are prescribed for people whose calcium levels get too high.

Anticonvulsants

Anticonvulsants are medications used to prevent seizures of any kind. Seizures occur when the electrical charges of the brain become disorganized. Epilepsy is the most common long-term seizure disorder. Anticonvulsants inhibit the repetitive spread of electrical impulses along nerve pathways. They also affect the liver's metabolism of vitamin D. When vitamin D isn't metabolized properly, the body doesn't absorb calcium very well. The most commonly used anticonvulsant is phenytoin (trade name, Dilantin ®). Phenobarbital, a less-used anticonvulsant, has the same effect. Since these drugs are taken for a lifetime, they should be supplemented with calcium and vitamin D.

Antacids

If you suffer from acid indigestion, gastric reflux disease, or ulcers you may be using an antacid for relief. Antacids work by neutralizing gastric acid secretions. Some antacids are salts derived from mineral sources, including calcium-robbing aluminum. Aluminum decreases the absorption of calcium and phosphate from the diet and increases calcium loss in the urine. Occasional use of these drugs is not a risk factor for osteoporosis, but abuse of aluminum based antacids can play a role in decreased bone density. Non-aluminum based antacids do not have this effect.

Aluminum Based Antacids	Non Aluminum Based Antacids
Aludros	Alka Seltzer
Amphojel	Bisodol
Gaviscon	Mylicon
Gelusil	*Rolaids
Kolantyl	*Titralac
Maalox	* Tums
Mylanta	
Riopan	

NOTE: this list is not intended to be a complete list of all aluminum containing antacids. Check with your pharmacist or look at the label on the product you use.

*These antacids contain calcium carbonate. Their supplemental use is beneficial to bones

Other Drugs Used Less Often

Lithium

One of the great advances in modern society is the acceptance that mental illnesses, which once sent us to institutions, or ostracized us from society, are biochemically based. Many mental illnesses can now be tempered with a combination of drugs and behavior therapy. One of these miracle drugs is Lithium. Lithium is used to treat manic depression, a syndrome marked by wide mood swings.

Lithium tempers these profound mental disturbances, but, like many drugs, it has side effects. In this case it is increased production of parathyroid hormone, which plays a role in the breakdown of bone. If Lithium has been prescribed for you, it is important that your mental health program include a physical activity program to keep your bones strong.

Anticancer Drugs

Drugs used to treat cancer prolong and save lives. They can also make bones fragile. It is not unusual for someone who is treated with these powerful medications for a long time to become vulnerable to fractures. Since these medications are crucial for survival and their benefits far outweigh the side effects they produce (and there are often many), there is very little interest in research to determine how these drugs harm bones. Sound nutrition and exercise, in keeping with physical stamina, are also an important part of treatment for cancer (or any disease). Keep the dialogue with your doctor open and be sure you are a partner in your treatment.

Heparin

Heparin is a blood thinner used to prevent or treat blood clots. It is rarely administered outside a hospital setting. People who need to take this injection daily, for a long time, have an increased risk of osteoporosis. Once again, the benefits of the drug far outweigh the risks.

What You Need to Know:

There are a variety of illnesses that call for a prescription or the recommendation of an over-the-counter medication that can contribute to weak bones. More often, these drugs aggravate an existing problem with osteoporosis, especially as we age and are likely to use more pills and potions on a regular basis. If you take any medicine for a long time, you need to ask your physician or pharmacist if the drugs that are helping you can also be harming your bones.

Chapter Seven

Your Sexual Lifestyle

"Bones and sex — what a great talk"!

Carol, Age 52

Can your sexual lifestyle really affect your bones?

Once you understand that sexual (reproductive) organs and sexual behavior (age menstrual periods begin, for example) depend on estrogen (and progesterone and testosterone) the "Can it?" becomes, "Yes, it can."

Periods Stopped for an Extended Time

Your menstrual period stops for a number of reasons. The most common are pregnancy and menopause. During these times there are tremendous fluctuations in sexual hormones. Some of these changes help bones (pregnancy) and some don't (menopause). However, other disturbances of the menstrual cycle are an important risk factor for osteopenia (low bone mass but not yet osteoporosis) and osteoporosis. Women who were amenorrheic (no periods) at any time are vulnerable to osteoporosis during their post-menopausal years.

Anorexia Nervosa and Bulimia

Although these eating conditions (described in Chapter 5) usually affect women, we don't know if they are or are not related to the sex hormones. One of the diagnostic criteria for anorexia is cessation of menses. Most long-term bulimics do not have normal menstrual cycles. If you don't eat, or if you binge and purge, your bones will suffer the consequences.

Female Athletes

Many competitive female athletes are amenorrheic. You would think that their high levels of physical training would overcome the low estrogen effects on their bones. It's not so. If these women are treated with hormone replacement therapy they maintain current bone mineral density but bone replacement does not occur. We've yet to meet a highly competitive athlete who makes osteoporosis prevention a higher priority than winning a race. They take their vitamins. They eat a healthy diet to improve performance. They also put themselves at risk for the development of hip or spinal compression fractures later in life. Don't get in their way with the osteoporosis prevention message. Understandably, their priorities are elsewhere.

Other Bone Makers and Bone Breakers

Disturbances of Ovulation

Women who have ovulatory disturbances without amenorrhea, meaning they have menstrual periods but do not ovulate, also have deficits in bone mass. These changes are not associated with excessive physical activity. Bone loss in these women is estimated to be 4.2 percent a year. The bone loss may be due to inadequate production of progesterone.

No Children

Women who have not given birth to children, by choice or because of fertility problems, seem to be at greater risk for osteoporosis. The reasons for this are not clear. It's possible they don't have the bone-building hormonal surges shared by women who experience pregnancy.

Late Menarche

Women who have an early onset of puberty and begin menstruating early have greater bone mass than women who begin menstruating in their late teens.

Hysterectomy

Pre-menopausal women who have a hysterectomy without removal of their ovaries have significantly lower bone density than normal menstruating women. It is not known if this bone loss is because the uterus was removed or the ovaries are, simply, no longer functioning properly.

Extended Lactation

Extended lactation (breastfeeding) is associated with bone loss. Typically, bone density improves and returns to pre-pregnancy levels within a year after a woman gives birth. When breastfeeding continues longer than a year, this return of bone density to pre-pregnancy levels does not occur. We don't know why this happens. Hopefully, new, safe drug strategies will emerge that can overcome a mother's desire to breastfeed her baby for a long time.

Early Menopause

As you already know, menopause is characterized by the loss of estrogen production by the ovaries. When menopause comes earlier than expected, whether it happens naturally (by age 45) or is induced by surgical removal of the ovaries, there are reduced levels of estrogen for a longer period of time than would occur with normal onset of menopause. Women whose ovaries are removed surgically can show signs of osteoporosis within two years if they do not receive hormone replacement therapy. That is why women who have early menopause and do not take HRT, are at increased risk for osteoporosis.

What Does Sexual Activity Have to Do with Bones?

In previous chapters you learned that a woman's bone mass reaches its peak around age 30-35, then it starts to decline. This is happening at the same time some women begin to have the decreased production of estrogen that becomes more pronounced during perimenopause and menopause.

You also learned about the role of alterable risk factors including weight bearing exercise on bone density. Well, what about sexual exercise? Don't be shocked. Author Beverly, who penned the best selling book, The G Spot, and more than eighty research articles about sexuality, reminds you that, depending on positions used during sexual intercourse, a woman can participate in weight bearing or non-weight bearing exercise with a loved one. Don't laugh! Sexual encounters are supposed to be good for you. This is your life. Be creative. Enjoy it. Think of, and use, intercourse positions that help provide weight bearing sexual activity and enjoyment for you and your lover.

Sexual Dysfunction and Your Bones

You may be surprised to learn that more than forty percent of women report a sexual problem at some time in their lives. The two most common are diminished sexual desire and a noticeable lack of lubrication. These two problems may be related to lower levels of estrogen in the body.

The decrease in vaginal lubrication may occur because as estrogen declines there is a reduced blood flow to the vagina. The wall of the vaginal lining becomes thinner and painful intercourse is the result. These changes may begin at the same time (the late 30s or 40s) as bone mass loss begins. Burning and pain during intercourse can begin long before a gynecologist is able to detect changes in the vagina. If this is a problem for you, use a water-based lubricant and consider hormone replacement therapy. Painful intercourse is not normal at any age. If you experience it, be sure to see your health-care provider.

A decrease in sexual desire can be related to other symptoms of perimenopause. When you are experiencing insomnia, night sweats, hot flashes, and irritability, a sexual lifestyle isn't a high priority. Hormone replacement therapy not only helps prevent osteoporosis, it also increases vaginal lubrication and sexual desire. Studies also support the message that women who masturbate or have intercourse regularly (that means once a week or more) have twice as much circulating estrogen as women who are not sexually active or active only sporadically. There's much to support the axiom, "Use it or lose it."

In short, you can have a healthy sexual life and prevent osteoporosis at the same time.

What You Need to Know:

Some of the sexual lifestyle choices that women make may affect their risk for osteoporosis. Any choice that decreases the amount of estrogen circulating in the body puts a woman at risk for osteoporosis. Having no children, extended breastfeeding, early menopause, or surgical menopause without HRT, are a few examples. An active sex life, including weight bearing sexual activity, is a good prescription for bone health.

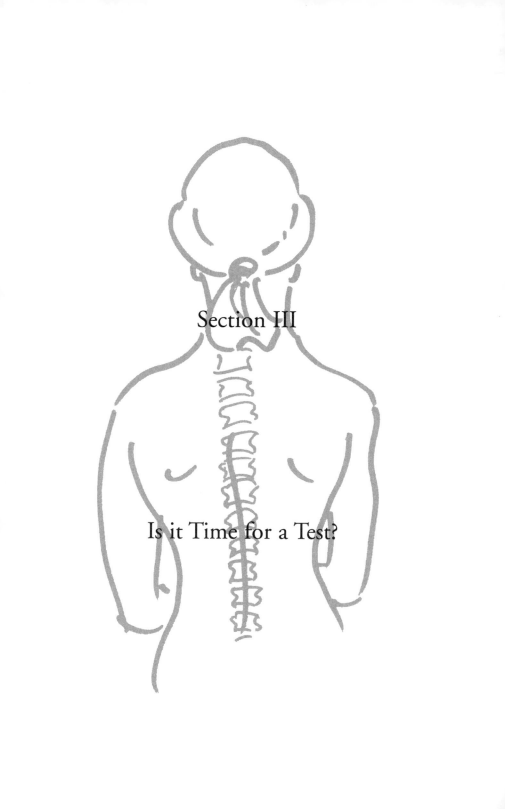

Section III

Is it Time for a Test?

"It never occurred to me to ask my doctor for a bone scan before my cancer chemotherapy. I'm spreading the word."
Sondra, Age 43

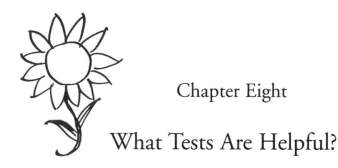

Chapter Eight

What Tests Are Helpful?

"Time to go beyond a heel scan to test my bones."
Nancy, Age 49

Too many women we meet worry about getting old. For many of them, aging means a less meaningful, less functional, and less productive life and the increased risk of poorer health that can accompany those extra birthday candles. This includes fear of osteoporosis. We believe this perspective is based on wearing the wrong color glasses to view the process of maturity.

When it comes to osteoporosis, read and repeat the following: "Deteriorating bones are not inevitable." Today's woman can prevent, and even reverse, bone loss by learning early, before you break a bone or shrink in height, if you are losing bone. All it takes is a visit to your doctor who, in most cases, will recommend you have tests to detect your risk for osteoporosis. With this information in hand, you and your health-care provider can make informed decisions regarding treatment of any existing disease and prevention of future bone loss. This is particularly important if you are struggling with a decision regarding the benefits and/or risks of hormone replacement therapy.

There are several useful and other not-so-useful tests to help this decision making process.

Tests that Don't Tell You What You Need to Know

Blood Tests (serum blood levels)

Most people have routine laboratory blood tests as part of their yearly physical. (Have you had yours this year? If not, call your gynecologist or primary physician today to schedule this vital review.) These blood tests are reported to your doctor as "serum blood levels." There are many assessments on this routine screen, including serum calcium and phosphorus. In addition, specialized laboratory tests, serum parathyroid hormone (PTH) and vitamin D metabolites, are often added if your medical history reveals a predisposition to osteoporosis.

Although the results of these tests can reveal red flags that signal a need for further tests or help a doctor identify osteoporosis in an already diagnosed case, osteoporosis cannot be diagnosed by a blood test. In fact, people with advancing osteoporosis can have normal blood tests, since the source of blood calcium is not revealed on serum blood level results. Nevertheless, blood tests may be useful in determining the cause of osteopenia (a decrease in bone density) or other disorders that cause changes in bone formation and breakdown.

X-ray studies

Although it seems logical that an x-ray that examines bone would help to establish a diagnosis of osteoporosis, that isn't the case. Approximately 30 to 50 percent of bone mass must be lost before the loss shows up on a routine x-ray.

Interestingly, slight overexposure of the x-ray film during processing may lead to the appearance of osteoporosis when it is not actually present.

Tests that Diagnose Osteoporosis

Bone Density Tests

The best tool for diagnosis (95 percent accurate) of brittle bones is called a bone-mineral-density (BMD) test. BMD testing can:

- establish the diagnosis of osteoporosis
- confirm the diagnosis in a person with a "fragility fracture"
- predict any future fracture risk
- monitor the progression of a diagnosed case of osteoporosis
- monitor the effects of therapy to halt or reverse osteoporosis

We agree with recommendation of The National Osteoporosis Foundation and other health organizations that recommend bone mineral density testing for:

- All postmenopausal women under age 65 who have at least one risk factor including: use of certain medications such as steroids or thyroid replacement therapy, eating disorders, a family history of osteoporosis, smoking, a small frame, excessive alcohol intake, poor diet, excessive dieting, and/or lifelong low calcium intake.
- All women over age 65.
- Postmemopausal women who have had a bone fracture.
- Women considering hormone replacement therapy (HRT) for whom a BMD would facilitate the decision.
- Women on HRT for a prolonged period of time.

> If you have any fracture be sure to ask your doctor for bone density evaluation.

Scoring BMD (Bone Mineral Density)

Whenever you take a test you get a score. The scoring system for BMD testing isn't the typical 0 – 100 system. Instead, a reference level is set based on optimum bone density for healthy young adults. The "standard" deviations (SD) from that norm, called T-scores, are given to the doctor of the individual being tested.

Low bone mass, termed osteopenia, is the diagnosis when a BMD reads between 1.0 and 2.5 SD below the mean. Osteoporosis is the diagnosis when a BMD reads 2.5 SD or more below the mean. If you have a score of 1 or more, you are not at risk for osteoporosis—today. If your score is between -1 and -2.5 this could indicate a risk for osteoporosis, but doesn't guarantee you have the disease—yet. A score of -2.5 or greater indicates bone loss of 25 percent or more. You will hear the bad news, "You have osteoporosis."

DEXA Scan

The preferred technique for measurement of bone density is the dual energy x-ray absorptiometry (DXA or DEXA). DEXA is the most widely used procedure for measuring bone density in clinical practice and research. The DEXA measures bone mineral density (BMD) in the spine, hip, or wrist, the most common sites for osteoporotic fractures. A DEXA scan requires no pills or injections and is painless. It can be completed in less than fifteen minutes with radiation exposure approximately one-tenth that of a standard chest x-ray.

If you are scheduled for this test you will be able to eat before you go, but will be instructed not to take a calcium supplement for 24 hours prior to the test. Some calcium supplements dissolve more slowly than others (more about that in Chapter 12). If yours is a slow absorbing variety, and some remains in your intestines when the DEXA is taken, you may get a false result.

When you arrive at the DEXA testing facility, you will be escorted into an "imaging" room. You will be asked a series of questions that review the risk factors for osteoporosis. Then you will be instructed to lie, fully clothed, on a padded table while the computerized scanner changes positions to record the necessary images.

A DEXA scan typically costs $100 to $500 or more, including the fee for the radiologist who interprets the scan. Nevertheless, it's the test of choice because its advantages far outweigh other, less expensive techniques. In 1994 there were 750 DEXA machines in the United States. As this book goes to press there are more than 4,000 machines in facilities nationwide.

> If you have a diagnosis of breast cancer put a DEXA scan near the top of your "to do" list. You can't afford to lose bone mass since estrogen replacement therapy is not one of your treatment options.

SXA Scan

Single-energy x-ray absorptiometry (SXA) and peripheral single-energy x-ray absorptiometry (pSXA) are techniques used to measure bone density in the forearm, finger, and heel. Because these screenings do not measure clinically relevant sites, they are not useful for diagnosis of osteoporosis. They are useful when assessing the bone density of some elderly people when calcification of bone interferes with DEXA test result accuracy.

Ultrasound

The FDA has recently approved ultrasound devices for bone density readings at the heel or other sites where bones are relatively close to the skin. These are the machines commonly seen at grocery stores, malls, and health conferences. Ultrasound testing can be helpful in screening for osteoporosis and to predict fracture risk. If you are scheduled for this test you will be asked to put your foot into a machine that takes measurements and provides results in minutes.

Ultrasound measurements are not as precise as DEXA or SXA, but appear to be able to predict fracture risk. These devices, which don't involve x-rays, are used in the doctor's office to flag women with very low bone density for further testing. They can help your doctor determine if you should have a DEXA scan. They do not make an accurate diagnosis of osteoporosis.

Other considerations

There is a direct correlation between BMD, as assessed by DEXA, and fracture risk. Bone size must also be considered in the assessment. Males do not have a greater BMD than females, but they do have bigger bones. Similarly, the advantage African-Americans have over Caucasians (they do not get osteoporosis as often) seems due to bigger bones rather than greater BMD.

WARNING: BMD accuracy can be impaired by poorly maintained equipment, patient movement, and coexisting disorders, such as degenerative joint disease.

Densitometry (DEXA) studies can also be used to monitor the effects of therapy in osteoporosis. The precision of measurement is very important in these circumstances. Repeat studies should be conducted at least every two years.

> Although doctors are becoming more savvy about the relationship between fractures and osteoporosis, a recent study of women over age 54 who suffered a wrist fracture revealed that only one-third were given a follow-up bone density scan to determine if the fracture was osteoporosis-related. If you break a bone be sure to ask your doctor, "Could this be an indication I'm at risk for osteoporosis?"

What You Need to Know

Eighty percent of low bone mass and osteoporosis goes unnoticed because, until recently, women weren't aware of testing options. **If you have any osteoporosis risk factors you should ask your health-care provider for a bone density test.** Heel scans, most commonly available to create awareness about this disease, can predict risk but the DEXA scan is the gold standard for diagnosing osteoporosis. Since many older women already have weak bones, be sure to ask your doctor to assess your risk compared to peak bone mass values in addition to those for women your age. Scoring is based on the results obtained from research on Caucasian women. Nevertheless, it is important for all women to be proactive. Don't panic if your bone density tests demonstrate your bones are as sturdy as a paper kite. There are new treatments to change the course of this disease.

Medicare will cover the cost for bone density tests every two years for people at risk and more frequently if medically necessary. The general medical coverage for BMD, according to the Bone Mass Measurement Act of 1998, includes: ·

- Estrogen-deficient woman at clinical risk for osteoporosis.
- A person with vertebral (spinal) abnormalities demonstrated by x-ray to indicate osteoporosis, low bone mass (osteopenia), or vertebral fracture.
- A person receiving, or expected to receive, a glucocorticoid therapy equivalent to 7.5 mg of prednisone or greater per day, for three months or more.
- A person with primary hyperparathyroidism.
- A person being monitored to assess her response to FDA-approved osteoporosis drug therapy.

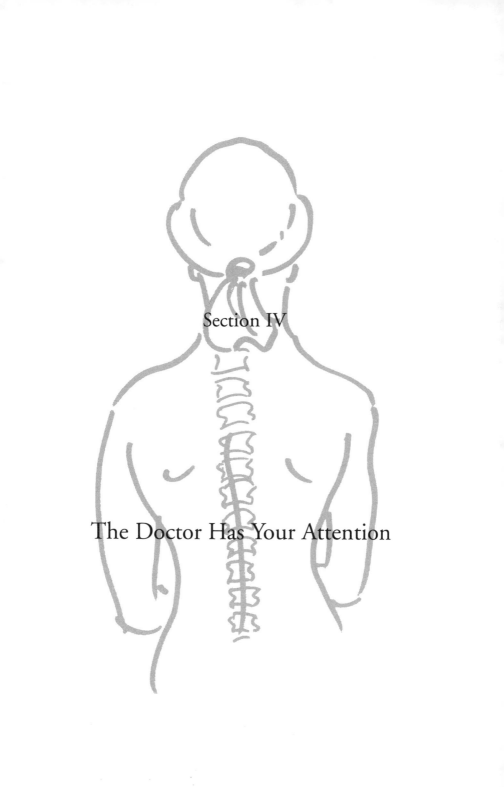

Section IV

The Doctor Has Your Attention

"I'm calling my doctor"

Too many to list

Chapter Nine

Treating Osteoporosis

"You convinced me - treating my osteoporosis will be the highest priority — no more skipped doses."

Mary, Age 71

If your bone scan results in a diagnosis of osteopenia or osteoporosis, the treatment prescribed for you will be determined by how far your disease has progressed.

- If you have not developed a critically low bone density, but are at increased risk for the development of osteoporosis, your focus will be on methods to prevent this disease.
- If you have a low bone mass (osteopenia), you will be encouraged to focus on methods of prevention with an emphasis on eliminating as many of the controllable risk factors as possible. (You can't change your gender or genetics.) Medication may also be added to the regimen.
- If a DEXA scan reveals you have osteoporosis, your treatment will be designed to prevent further bone loss, increase bone mass, and prevent fractures. This will probably include medication.

• If you already have fractures and deformities, you may also be prescribed drugs and/or treatments to relieve pain, in addition to medication to treat your disease.

Stage	Goal
At risk for the development of osteoporosis	Prevent bone loss; maintain bone strength
Low bone density but no fractures	Prevent further bone loss; increase bone mass; prevent fractures
Low bone density and fractures	Prevent further bone loss; increase bone mass; prevent further fractures;relieve pain
Osteoporosis with disability	Prevent further bone loss; increase bone mass; prevent further fractures; relieve pain; rehabilitation services

Medications For Treatment

Have you ever gone to pick up a prescription and been stunned by the cost? Before you get upset with your pharmacist, consider that there is much more factored into the cost of that prescription than the medicine itself. In fact, you are paying for the research and development that went into developing the drug, the testing that assured its safety, the purchase, processing, packaging of the drug in a proper environment, the marketing required to make published research available to physicians and other health-care providers, the shipping to the dispensing pharmacy, the cost of storage, salaries for staff, rent for the building, and so on. Perhaps you are not aware of the billions spent by companies developing medications that are never proven effective enough to make it to market. When one of these ventures is successful we get some wonderful products that improve our length and quality of life-including the new drugs that are a critical part of the strategies for treating osteoporosis.

Drug interventions currently approved to prevent and treat osteoporosis include: estrogen, SERMS, bisphosphonates, calcitonin, and the supplements, calcium, and vitamin D.

Estrogen

Estrogen was first indicated for the treatment of post-menopausal osteoporosis only. Now the FDA supports the use of estrogen for the prevention of osteoporosis and as part of the management of established osteoporosis. These drugs work by inhibiting bone resorption, although the mechanism of action is not clear.

When estrogen is prescribed it is described in two ways:
• Hormone replacement therapy (HRT) indicates the medication includes estrogen AND progesterone.
• Estrogen replacement therapy (ERT) indicates the medication includes only estrogen. Since there is a risk of cancer of the uterus when progesterone is not included in therapy, this drug strategy is used only in women who no longer have a uterus.

Estrogens act to maintain or increase bone mineral density (BMD) by approximately one to three percent. This effect may occur even when menopause occurred up to 10 years earlier, but it is greatest when hormone replacement therapy is started within the first five years after menopause. If you are given a prescription for HRT, you can expect to take it for the rest of your life.

There are many estrogen products available by prescription. They come in pills and patches. Only some of them have been approved for treatment of osteoporosis. They include:

Conjugated equine estrogen, 0.625 mg (Premarin®)

17 beta-Estradiol transdermal patches, 0.05 mg (Estraderm®)

Transdermal estrogen patch (Vivelle®)

Piperazine estrone sulfate, 0.75 mg (Ogen®)

Esterfied estrogens, 0.3 mg, 0.625 mg, and 2.5 mg (Estratab®)

Five years of HRT decreases spinal fractures by 50 to 80 percent and other fractures, including hip and wrist, by approximately 25 percent.

Other Effects of Estrogen
In addition to protecting you from osteoporosis, estrogens may have a beneficial effect on your heart and may help with Alzheimer's type of dementia. The drawback is that long-term use of estrogen (more than 5-10 years) increases your risk for breast cancer (30-35 percent). Deaths from heart

attacks and complications from osteoporosis generally outweigh the risks for breast cancer in the general population. However, for women with high risk of breast cancer and low risk of heart disease, this is not the case. These women MUST weigh the benefits and risks of ERT with her physician.

Women on ERT may be predisposed to blood clots in the deep veins of the leg. These kind of clots can "break loose" and cause a deadly blockage in the lungs called a pulmonary embolism. Once again, risk analysis is required.

Compliance With Estrogen Therapy

Despite the beneficial effects of ERT/HRT on the skeleton and on other systems and the recommendation that they be continued throughout life, few women comply with this recommendation. The reasons for this are complex and cultural and include an aversion to taking pills and the concerns about breast cancer described above. The sad outcome of this is that women who stop taking estrogen begin to lose bone density until, after age 75, it is the same as if they hadn't used the drug at all. What most women don't realize is that the amount of estrogen in ERT/HRT is much less than the amount in birth control pills they may have taken for years.

Estrogen may be one of the most useful post-menopausal medications women can use. Despite its obvious and proven benefits, the long-term effects, including the risk of breast and endometrial cancer, have made its use controversial. In the case of endometrial cancer, the risk can be reduced by adding progesterone, which also seems to promote bone formation and increase bone turnover. Adding progesterone to estrogen therapy (becoming HRT vs. ERT) is standard practice for women who have a uterus and have gone through natural menopause. However, progesterone also produces side effects, including a predisposition to blood clots, so some women feel they can't win. Nevertheless, and we can't say it loudly enough, don't discard estrogen as an option for continuing good health until you weigh all the risks and benefits. Work with your health-care provider and a compounding pharmacist until you have the lowest dose that gives the benefits you deserve.

Although the decision to take estrogen replacement therapy is an individual one, most doctors suggest that women who can take estrogen, do so. In addition to maintaining bone density, estrogen also protects the cardiovascular system and may decrease the risk of heart attack and stroke.

A Selective Estrogen Receptor Modulator (SERM)

There is a new class of drugs called Selective Estrogen Receptor Modulators (SERMS). Some people refer to them as "designer estrogens." SERMS are not hormones but act like the hormone, estrogen, in many ways. Raloxifene (Evista® by Lilly & Co.) was introduced in 1997 after it was approved by the FDA for the prevention, but not the treatment, of osteoporosis. New studies showed it reduces the risk of spinal fracture by about half, so it has received approval to treat the disease. Unlike estrogen, Evista® does not appear to be associated with the increased risk of vaginal bleeding or breast or uterine cancer. An additional benefit is its positive effect on the cardiovascular system because it lowers blood levels of cholesterol. It is not without side effects. Evista® has been known to cause blood clots and hot flashes.

Bisphosphonates

When you get a ring around your bathtub or in your toilet bowl there are cleaners that magically dissolve this mineral "scum." In essence, the chemicals in the cleaner attach themselves to the mineral and make it easy to be washed away. Similar "chemicals" soften hard water and prevent the lime (calcium) deposits that make our porcelain fixtures look so dirty.

These same chemicals, called bisphosphonates, love calcium so much that when they are taken orally they rush to your bones where they prevent bone-breaking osteoclasts from doing their job (See Chapter 3). As a drug, bisphosphonates increase bone mineral density and reduce the incidence of spinal fractures and the potentially devastating fracture of the hip.

In chapter six you learned that sometimes a gain/loss benefit must be weighed when a patient is given a medication. That is why taking a potent, but helpful drug, like one of the corticosteroids, is used despite the possibility it can cause drug induced osteoporosis. A bisphosphonate is the drug of choice for women who have an underlying disease that requires them to be on these bone-robbing steroids for a long period of time.

There are two potent bisphosphonates approved for use in the USA to prevent and treat osteoporosis. The first one released was alendronate (Fosamax® by Merck & Co.). In controlled clinical trials alendronate reduced the incidence of fracture at the spine, hip, and wrists by 50 percent in women with osteoporosis. Women with fractures of their vertebrae who used this drug had fewer days of limited activity. However, there have been problems with this medication because there are potential side effects such as upper gastrointestinal disturbances, heartburn, painful or difficulty swallowing and gastric reflux. That is why, if Fosamax® is prescribed for you, you will be given very specific instructions about how the drug should be taken. You must take your pill first thing in the morning at least 30 minutes before you eat or drink anything else because food and liquids (except water) easily interfere with the absorption of Fosamax®. You will also be told to remain upright for the first 30 minutes after you take the medicine to prevent any reflux that can irritate the esophagus. Prescriptions work best when they are used as directed. This is especially true of drugs that are used to reverse life-threatening silent diseases like osteoporosis.

> It is very important to take a bisphosphonate as directed on the package to avoid digestive problems.

The Newest Bisphosphonate

In April, 2000, the FDA approved the newest drug in the bisphosphonate market. Risedronate (Actonel®, by Procter & Gamble Pharmaceuticals and Aventis Pharmaceuticals) is a treatment for osteoporosis that has captured the attention of doctors. Actonel® increases bone mass, stops bone loss, and produces healthy bone in women with established postmenopausal osteoporosis. In recent studies, patients who used this drug had a significant reduction in new spinal and non-spinal fractures. Actonel has also been shown to reduce the risk of hip fracture in women with confirmed osteoporosis. In addition, research revealed there is a rapid, one year benefit of decreased risk of vertebral fractures with Actonel® that was not seen with earlier bisphosphonates. Use of this treatment comes with dosage instructions similar to earlier bisphosphonates. Research studies show any side effects are the same as those reported by women receiving a placebo.

> Anytime you experience discomfort after using any medication you should let your doctor know immediately before making a decision to continue or discontinue using the drug.

Calcitonin

Sometimes when something mimics the action of something else it acquires a name that sounds like the original name. This is the case with calcitonin, which sounds like calcium—its partner in your body. Calcitonin is a hormone made by your thyroid gland, which monitors how much calcium is in your blood. If blood calcium levels get high, calcitonin will get things back to normal by decreasing the number and activity of the osteoclasts. That prevents bone calcium from leaving the bone and returns calcium already in the blood to the bone, which helps increase bone mass. In other words calcitonin adds calcium to your bones when there are high blood calcium levels.

When researchers are looking for new ways of treating disease they often look to animals to find out if the animals have the same biochemicals that humans do. That kind of research revealed that many animals have calcitonin. Further research revealed that salmon calcitonin was the best variety to treat osteoporosis. Now, pharmacological preparations of both synthetic human and salmon calcitonin are available, but only salmon calcitonin has been FDA approved for osteoporosis treatment.

Calcitonin is indicated for the treatment of osteoporosis in women who are more than five years post-menopause, have a low BMD, and are not candidates for estrogen treatment. It is available for injection (Calcimar® by Rhone-Poulenc Rorer or Miacalcin® by Sandoz) or the more popular nasal spray (Miacalcin®) that is rapidly absorbed through the tissues in your nose. If you are given a prescription for the nasal spray, each daily spray will deliver 200 units of the drug. Calcitonin can reduce the risk of spinal fractures by 40 percent, but it doesn't work as well on other bones.

Salmon calcitonin is one of the safest of the drugs available for the treatment of osteoporosis. An advantage of its use is that it also relieves the pain of osteoporosis. Drawbacks are nasal irritation and bleeding.

If you are taking a prescription drug designed to decrease your fracture risk, don't neglect to also meet daily requirements for calcium and vitamin D to assure you receive optimal treatment results.

Fluoride

When you hear the word fluoride, you probably think "teeth." You should also think "bones." Health sleuths are always observing the changes that occur when a chemical is used in any situation. In the case of fluoride, a lower incidence of osteoporosis in areas where there was lots of fluoride in the water made scientists sit up and take notice. A well planned research study revealed this truth: drink fluoridated water and you will have more bone density than women who don't. This increase occurs mostly in trabecular and some corticol bone. As is often the case with research, they still haven't ferreted out the hows and whys of the change. They are unclear about the quality of that new bone, which in some studies showed increased bone mass but decreased bone strength. Regardless, it's an important finding.

Fluoride treatment of osteoporosis in the United States has reached an impasse. The studies regarding the success of its use have been dramatic but they have been small. There are a couple of combinations of slow release fluoride combined with calcium citrate being used in Europe, but the jury is still out in the United States.

Calcium and Vitamin D

It is now common knowledge that calcium supplements can help prevent osteoporosis. We still don't know how effective they are for the treatment of osteoporosis because the effects of calcium supplementation on fracture rates have been inconsistent.

The best use of calcium in the treatment of osteoporosis may be its ability to improve the effects of other drugs. This is good because any time you take a prescription you want to use the lowest dose possible to get the desired result. That is why most clinical trials of osteoporosis now include calcium supplements and many add vitamin D.

Women at risk for osteoporosis, especially elderly women who often don't eat properly, should be sure that they have an adequate calcium intake. You will learn more about the importance of calcium for general nutrition and for supporting optimum skeletal growth in adolescents in Chapters 12 and 13.

You get your best bang for your calcium buck when you divide your daily intake of calcium supplement into at least two doses and take it with food and lots of water. Multiple doses encourage efficient absorption. Calcium supplements should not be taken with caffeine, iron, or fiber products because they bind the calcium and prevent absorption in your GI tract. There are many forms of calcium supplements. The more expensive, soluble salts, like calcium citrate, are better absorbed so they are worth the extra money in the long run. Check out Chapter 13 for more in-depth information about calcium supplementation.

You can do a mini-science experiment in your kitchen. Check the speed at which your calcium will be absorbed by putting a tablet in a half cup of vinegar. The goal is to have the tablet disintegrate, not disappear, within one half-hour. Speed of absorption in the vinegar, which mimics stomach acids,

indicates speed of absorption in your GI tract. Never knew
how easy it was to be a scientist, did you?

Emerging Treatments

Several new therapies are under study for the prevention
and treatment of osteoporosis. They include other SERMS,
growth hormone, parathyroid hormone, statin drugs, and
non-loop diuretics.

Anabolic steroids promote bone formation, but their use
in women is limited by their virilizing effects (and in men by the
harmful effects on the cardiovascular system and prostate). Our
friend, Dr. Robert Lindsay, who wrote the foreword of this
book, encourages us to mention exciting research with parathyroid hormone, which not only prevented post-menopausal
bone loss but also increased bone mass density in the spine.

Another study showed that hydrochlothiazide, a
common diuretic that is not in the category of "loop diuretics"
that can cause bone loss, preserved bone density at the hip and
spine over a three-year period when compared to a placebo.
The benefit, though modest, was well tolerated making the
drug a consideration in programs to prevent osteoporosis-
especially in women who need to take diuretics.

The aggressive research currently being conducted seems
certain to provide additional effective drugs to prevent or end
bone loss or rebuild bone. We are indeed encouraged that our
premise that living long can mean living well is a reality for
smart women everywhere.

Alternative Therapies

The media has given lots of publicity to several alternative therapies. These include growth hormone, DHEA, and
phytoestrogens. Growth hormone is beneficial in calcium
deficient children and adults, but it is not indicated for osteo-

porosis. There is no scientific evidence that DHEA has any efficacy in the management of osteoporosis. Soy is a plant estrogen or phytoestrogen. Researchers at the University of Illinois discovered that post-menopausal women who were on a soy diet for six months had a increase in (only) spinal bone density. Nevertheless, most osteoporosis specialists believe phytoestrogens are not powerful enough to be useful in the treatment of osteoporosis. More research is needed on all these and other alternative therapies that are sure to emerge as our population ages. Osteoporosis is a serious disease. We agree with physicians who urge women to stick with medicine that has been proven, by science, to work.

There is evidence that both estrogen and androgens have some role in maintaining bone mass in both genders. However, there is no evidence that estrogen treatment for men with osteoporosis or androgen treatment for women with osteoporosis is effective and the side effects and safety concerns of these reverse regimens don't warrant their use.

What You Need to Know:

There are now many types of medication available to treat osteoporosis. If you are diagnosed with this disease you need to discuss the treatment options with your physician. Unless you have a personal or family history of breast cancer your doctor may recommend a drug combination of estrogen and progesterone. If you have had your uterus removed you don't need the progesterone. The "designer estrogens" known as SERMS (Evista®) are not contraindicated when there is breast cancer risk. The bisphosphonates (such as Fosamax® and the recently approved Actonel®) and calcitonin (Miacalcin®) stop or slow bone breakdown, prevent bone loss, and actually increase bone mass in osteoporotic women (and men). Calcium and vitamin D help maintain bone mass and are essential in any treatment of osteoporosis. If you are diagnosed with osteoporosis you need to discuss the treatment options, consider how your body responds to the choices made, then commit to and stick with the regimen that is the best fit for managing your disease and improving your bone health. Since failure to comply with doctor's orders can have serious consequences it is imperative you develop a routine that assures you "take your medicine" every day.

Don't fall into the trap of believing that because you are taking a bone-building prescription drug you don't need to continue to take a calcium and vitamin D supplement and eat a high in calcium diet. This assures optimal treatment results.

Don't panic if you are diagnosed with osteoporosis, are given a prescription, take it regularly, but fail to get an increase in bone density right away. Stick with your program. Persistance and patience are the key to the treatment of this disease. Improvement can occur.

Remember, you and your health-care provider are PARTNERS in the decision as to what treatment strategies are best for you.

Chapter Ten

Physical Activity Builds Strong Bones

"Thanks for clarifying what 'weight bearing exercise' means."

Sandi, Age 55

Suppose, after reading this book, you have a DEXA scan that reveals you have osteoporosis. Or, in a worst case scenario, you have a simple fall that results in a not so simple fracture. Perhaps, like too many of our older friends, a simple movement causes such severe back pain you call your doctor, who orders x-rays that show you have one or more spontaneous fractures in your spine.

The treatment outlined for you will take into consideration all the factors outlined in earlier chapters of this book. Whether that regimen includes estrogen, bisphosphonates, calcitonin, or supplements, you can pretty much count on a suggestion to exercise. If you already have an exercise strategy in place, it may, or may not, need to be modified to support the changes in bone density exercise provides. If exercise has not been a part of your lifestyle, the instruction to exercise may have little meaning for you. How do you begin? What's the best kind?

Exercise, for the purpose of treating osteoporosis includes two kinds of activities:
1. **aerobic exercise on a hard surface**
2. **anaerobic exercise that strengthens muscle**

We believe it is essential to understand the principles underlying good advice. For the purpose of exercise this includes basic knowledge about how your body works. Armed with this information you can make the best individual decision about which exercise program is the wisest choice for your overall good health, including the strength and density of your bones. So, bear with us while we talk "physiology."

Exercise professionals distinguish the differences between aerobic and anaerobic exercise based on the physiological requirements for fuel in the muscles you use when you "work out."

Fuel to Support Bone Building Exercise

Like a car, your muscles require fuel to work. You don't get to choose which fuel will be used. All you can do is eat as healthfully as possible, store the energy the food provides, and wait for a muscle to choose the fuel that is best for the work at hand. These muscle fuels are either sugar, in the form of glucose, or fat in the form of fatty acids. The sugar comes from the carbohydrates you eat—the fresh fruits, vegetables, and whole grains, as well as sugars you add to foods. The fat comes from the fat you eat—that already present in meat, milk, and milk products, as well as any fat you add to foods. You also eat protein—in meat, milk, and the scant amounts found in fruits, vegetables, and grains. However, muscles don't like protein very much for muscle work. They prefer to use the protein after the workout, when they respond to your effort by becoming stronger.

Macronutrient/Fuel	Is In These Foods
Carbohydrates	fruits, vegetables, whole grains + empty calorie added sugars
Fat	meat, whole milk and whole milk products, added fats like butter, margarine, salad dressings
Protein	meat, poultry, fish, milk and milk products (choose low fat), eggs

Regardless of your food choice, carbohydrate, fat, or protein, food is a source of energy that is measured in calories. Some of that caloric energy is used right away. Any extra is stored in your body until you need it. Some of us have too much stored energy. The only advantage to this abundant storage, which we call "being overweight," is that overweight people often have stronger bones to support that extra weight. If you are overweight you may be happy to hear this news. Before you get too excited, remember, the many health consequences of being overweight far outweigh this single advantage.

Aerobic Exercise

The word aerobic means "with oxygen." From the perspective of exercise physiology, aerobic exercise is an activity that requires the presence of oxygen in the muscle cell in order to convert stored fat (energy) to fuel for muscle work. Normal activities, including sleeping, eating, and walking around, are aerobic. Even when you are exercising so intensely that you get out of breath there is some aerobic activity in the muscle. For the purpose of treating bones, your aerobic activity must force your heart and lungs to work harder than normal but not so hard that you get out of breath. Typically the activity uses the big muscles of the lower body for a sufficient amount of time, and often enough, to gain benefits.

The program you choose can be varied in three ways. There's an acronym that makes this easy to understand. It's FIT where:

F = frequency, or how often you exercise
I = intensity, or how hard you exercise
T = time, or how long you exercise

You have a choice to:

1. **Exercise frequently, but not hard or for very long**
2. **Exercise with "intensity," so you don't have to exercise as often or as long**
3. **Exercise for a long time so you don't have to exercise as often or as hard**

Of course, you can combine these three variables in various ways. In fact, your results will be based on how many of the variables are brought into play. If you exercise often, hard, and for long periods of time you are more prone to injury. If you exercise rarely, at a low intensity, and for short periods of time, it will be a long time before you see results. As in most things, moderation is the best course of action.

Some exercise specialists add a second T (for technique) to describe the kind of exercise you choose. For the purpose of treating osteoporosis, this is "weight bearing" exercise. Weight bearing exercise means there is a lot of your weight on the exercising surface. That could include walking, dancing, playing tennis, climbing stairs, or anything else that creates an impact on a floor, stair, track, or street surface.

Aerobic exercise will warm your body and make more than your bones fit, because it is systemic. A systemic exercise means major or big muscles are being used in ways that effect change all over your body.

If you exercise at this FREQUENCY	And your INTENSITY is	The suggested amount of TIME of the exercise session	For this Suggested TECHNIQUE
2-3 x day	low to moderate	10-15 minutes	walk, low impact aerobics, exercise machine
Daily	moderate to hard	30-40 minute	jog/run, step aerobics
Daily	low to moderate	60-90 minutes	walk

Aerobic Exercise Is Systemic

Suppose you stood up and, holding on to a chair, bent your knee and lifted your leg up, then down, repeatedly. After a while the muscles lifting your leg might get tired, but chances are you wouldn't get warm from the effort. You might argue that the exercise is aerobic because you are standing. You are even using big muscles in the lower body. But, since the effort is so localized to the muscle in the upper leg, other body systems don't work very hard. Suppose, instead, you sat in a chair, then stood up and sat down ten or twenty times.

Chances are you would start to get breathless and warm because so many muscles are being used. That is (systemic) aerobic exercise. Standing up and sitting back down is good aerobic exercise because the big muscles of the lower body are being used, but, once again, to help bones the goal is impact. Keep thinking, "grow, osteoblasts, grow."

How Hard Should Aerobic Weight Bearing Exercise Be?
    As for intensity, ignore the formulas that take your age into consideration. Your current fitness level is the determining factor in setting exercise pace, not your age. That pace should be hard enough to make you slightly breathless while you exercise but not hard enough to leave you gasping for breath. Pay attention to how you feel as you exercise. On a good day, when your routine is comfortable and you feel safe, push yourself a little harder. If you don't feel up to par another day, take it easy, but KEEP DOING SOMETHING. There are many days when your authors do not want to exercise. We operate with the following philosophy: The first day we don't exercise is the first day of poor habit building we will regret later. Besides, after we get our blood pumping and get back home, we are ALWAYS glad we put in the effort.

Anaerobic Exercise

    The second type of exercise is anaerobic exercise. If aerobic means with oxygen, anaerobic means without oxygen. That may sound silly, because you never stop breathing when you exercise. But when you do an exercise so intensely you can't deliver enough oxygen to the muscle to burn fat for fuel, the muscle will call on a different energy supply that burns fuel without using oxygen. That fuel is stored sugar, called glycogen, which quickly converts to the simple sugar (glucose) that muscles can burn.

Anaerobic exercise happens in two ways. One is by exercising so hard you become breathless. When you exercise hard, rest briefly, repeat the effort, then rest again, you are interval training. Your muscles respond to these "intervals" in the same way your bones respond to the continuing effort of aerobic exercise. They get more fit. The other kind of anaerobic exercise is built around strength training. Sometimes this is called resistance training, weight training, or body-building. It is, simply, any exercise that makes a muscle stronger, larger, and more dense.

Until recently, anaerobic exercise didn't get the respect it deserves. Sure, women could get more fit and stronger with anaerobic exercise but few of us sprint or lift or push the excessively heavy items that warranted training for that kind of effort.

Now we know anaerobic exercise, or strength training, is a superior way to treat and prevent osteoporosis. Think of a slingshot. It has a forked stick with a thick rubber band attached to it. The strength of the stick determines how much force you're able to put on the band to sling your rock. If the stick is strong it will withstand a lot of force. The same is true of the relationship between your muscle and bones. Your bone has a distinct advantage over the stick. It can get stronger as the muscle "bands" attached become stronger. When you strengthen your muscles you not only strengthen bones you are preventing falls.

> Your goal for strength training the lower body is to be able to get up from a chair without using your arms to give you an added push.

There's another advantage to strengthening muscles that may motivate you to get started (or keep you interested) in anaerobic exercise. Building muscle is an extraordinary metabolism booster. When your metabolism is fast you burn more calories per minute than a person whose metabolism is slow, whether you are sitting around or working out. In other words, the more muscle you have, the more calories you burn per minute.

The aerobic exercise and anaerobic strength training strategies designed to treat osteoporosis are pretty much the same as methods used to prevent osteoporosis. (See Chapter 14.) If you are just beginning an exercise program there are some guidelines, designed especially for beginners, to help you make a smart start.

Your Exercise Program

1. Find an exercise you enjoy. Better yet, find several exercises you enjoy—or at least find tolerable. That's the only way to assure you'll keep coming back for more. We encourage beginners to look back to their childhood and remember what activities they enjoyed. Repeat them as an adult, and your heart will sing again. When adult Ronda got on a bicycle with upright handlebars, similar to those on the bike she had in her youth, she rediscovered a passion for cycling she'd never experienced stooped over on the touring bicycle she'd used for years.

One of the more popular theories in the exercise movement today is called cross-training or cross-conditioning. When you do several kinds of exercise you use many different muscle groups. You are less likely to be injured. Cross-training is also good to create alternatives when the weather is bad or you are away from your regular exercise routine. Consider buying a couple of exercise videos (see resources in our appendix) to use when you have no alternative but to exercise at home.

2. Start slowly. This guideline is about injury prevention. You may be enthusiastic and want to conquer this disease as soon as possible, but Rome wasn't built in a day. Neither is a fit and strong body. Your effort should progress until you are moving longer, more often, and with sufficient intensity to help those bones.

Since almost everyone walks, a graduated walking program is a good place to begin. (See the appendix in the back of this book for a walking program that has helped many people move from not so fit bones to stronger bones in a relatively short period of time.) Walk alone or walk with friends. Use our guidelines (page 157) to assure you get the best out of your effort to support stronger bones without a risk of injury.

3. Be patient. Adults are so impatient. We spend a lot of time teaching children patience, then neglect the lesson ourselves. Instead of attempting to whip yourself into shape in a few short weeks, progress slowly. You will add another dimension of injury prevention, which will leave you saying, "Hmmm...that wasn't so bad; maybe tomorrow I'll go a little farther or faster or longer." Until recently, intensity was put on the back burner of an exercise program since so many people were hurt when they worked out too hard. Now we have good shoes and safer exercise surfaces that allow us to focus on intensity and get fit fast. Still, it's not the best way to go if you are a beginner.

4. Exercise often. You get the real benefits of exercise when you do it consistently. Essentially, you remind your muscles this activity is going to happen on a regular basis and they become more efficient at utilizing stored fuel. If you are an absolute beginner, you're better off exercising for short periods of time several times a day. If this time frame doesn't work for you, exercise for at least 20-30 minutes, a minimum of four times a week. You can sustain a current fitness level working out two to three times a week, but you will need to exercise more often for bone-building results.

5. Do ANYTHING that will help you stick with your program. Set short- and long-term goals that will motivate, not discourage you. Some people like the structure of a planned program, and record keeping helps them to measure their goals. Other people like to go with the flow and decide what they are going to do, and when, on a daily basis.

There's no right time to exercise. Studies have been conducted that show exercise in the morning keeps your metabolism high all day, while exercise in the evening burns more calories when you sleep. Instead of worrying about which choice will give you the best bang for your buck, exercise at the time of day that assures you will stick with your program.

If you're lucky, your doctor will refer you to a physical therapist or exercise physiologist who can evaluate your current fitness level and get you started on the right foot (if you'll excuse the pun). Personal trainers, working independently or in health clubs, enjoy designing programs customized to your current level of fitness, needs, and goals. For those of you who don't have that luxury, you can still blast your osteoblasts into a higher level of production, and discourage the osteoclasts from doing their bone breaking work, with a self-designed program you enjoy. Our mantra: "Smart women who exercise have strong bones."

What You Need to Know:

Any sound strategy to combat osteoporosis should begin with a solid aerobics program that focuses on weight bearing exercises like walking, jogging, stair-stepping, tennis, dance, or step aerobics. In addition, you should engage in a strength building program (lift weights) for both the upper and lower body to increase bone strength and get the added value of a boosted metabolism. Use of the acronym FITT where F = frequency, I = intensity, T = time, and T = technique, can help assure you will put forth enough effort to gain the kind of fitness results that help maintain bone density. Your exercise regimen should be designed around activities you enjoy, start and build slowly to prevent injury and maintain motivation, and be repeated often enough to remind your body this new program is a lifetime effort.

Chapter Eleven

Identifying and Using Support

"Support groups for our support structure — I'm calling NOF tomorrow,"

Michelle, Age 64

Easy for us to say, "Just do it." In fact, keeping motivated is one of the toughest dilemmas for people who choose to alter their life. So, what can we offer you to help you "Stick with it?"

First, let's look at success. There are two industries (so to speak) that are pros at providing support. For more than seventy years 12-step recovery programs have been a force behind life changes for people whose lives were perilously threatened by addictions to substances (drugs, alcohol, food) or processes (gambling, shopping, relationships). The 12-step model has been adapted so widely that there are now support groups for almost anything. The weight loss industry has also moved from "just do it," to programming that provides counseling and support to clients. Interestingly, the fastest growing successful weight loss programs are not commercial programs.

They are in religious communities where men and women gather to fill themselves with spirit and love of God instead of the love of food. Why do these programs work?

Anytime you make a change, you have an internal psychological support system that is used to the way you live your life. People content with your current way of life surround you. Modify your lifestyle and, unless the rewards are great, patterns deeply embedded in your subconscious can become an obstacle to your new lifestyle. The people you live and work with may give lip service to your lifestyle change, especially when it is "good for you," but they might also, consciously or subconsciously, sabotage your effort if it means they also have to change.

Support Groups

There are support groups springing up nationwide for people with osteoporosis. You can gather with people who share your disease and recovery to help problem solve any dilemma that may rear its ugly head. Typically, a support group will invite guest speakers, distribute educational materials, and share gossip regarding which doctors and treatments give good results. The best resource is your local osteoporosis center or the office of a physician whose treatment specialty includes osteoporosis. The National Osteoporosis Foundation keeps an ongoing list of these ever-changing support groups. It also provides guidelines to help start one. Their contact number and web site address are on page 148 in the appendix of this book.

Internet

The Internet is filled with resources for learning more about osteoporosis, medications that treat the disease, and information about exercise programming.

http://www.swh.net or http://www.speakingofwomen-shealth.com is a good place to start. This reliable resource is jam packed with useful information, archived presentations by some of the best speakers on women's health issues, and practical strategies to keep you smart. Beyond that, all you need to do is use a search engine and type in the word "osteoporosis," or a drug name, or the word "exercise." If you use the Internet frequently, you probably have a favorite search engine, but each one lists different resources, so try several to give you more results. There are also chat groups and newsgroups where you can meet people who share your interests and give you immediate feedback and support. Your Internet provider probably has an extensive list of chat groups. Our search of the Internet also located individual web sites created by people who have their own resource lists for learning more about osteoporosis. Because these resources change so rapidly your best bet is to do your own search, or ask your librarian to do one for you.

These resources come with a caveat: "User beware." In addition to the many reputable people, agencies, and associations willing to help you, there are unscrupulous people who may give you false information or attempt to sell you something that may not be useful or wise for you to use. The Internet can be a great resource for value when it comes to supplements or prescriptions but remember, these drugs can react with other supplements and prescriptions. If you are on a prescription drug you shouldn't add anything to your regimen without checking with your doctor. Your pharmacist is your best resource for discussing drug interactions. Guidelines about supplement use are in Chapter 13.

Psychological Support

The psychological issues that can emerge when you or someone in your family has chronic pain or illness can be overwhelming. Sure, you can sweat it out on your own and pull yourself up by the bootstraps, or you can yield, admit you aren't coping as well as you hoped, and get some professional help. If your disease challenges your mental health, don't fail to seek professional counseling to help you deal with any changes you must make. The coping skills and attitude adjustments that result from the wise counsel of a professional are well worth your time and money. Interview your prospective mental health professional with the same care you would take to interview a specialist of any kind. Pay attention to gut feelings about the professional as well as the setting where the counseling is offered. Ask others in the same boat if they have a professional they know and trust. The acknowledgment that psychological strategies can support the prevention and treatment of disease is one of the great breakthroughs in the medical profession. Take advantage of it.

What You Need to Know:

One factor highly correlated with successful change is good support. Typically this involves family and friends, but can extend to professional assistance or peer-related groups and support agencies, including those that focus on helping people with osteoporosis.

When you make a mutual commitment to give and receive support with others, you will find the encouragement, education, and understanding to help you through many rough spots you may encounter in the treatment of your bone health.

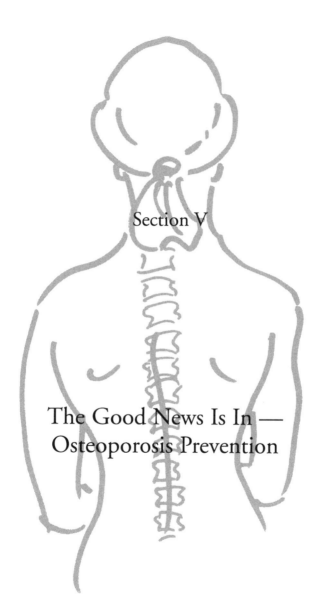

Section V

The Good News Is In —
Osteoporosis Prevention

"I didn't realize how much I could do to prevent osteoporosis."

Ruth Ellen, Age 18

Chapter Twelve

Proper Diet

"My children will get milk everyday"

Debi, Age 35

Osteoporosis is preventable. Thanks to science we continue to identify causes and improve methods for diagnosis and treatment. In this edition we can say, unequivocally, that the ravages of this devastating disease-brittle bones, unnecessary fracture's, and dowager's humps can be tempered in our lifetime and eliminated in future generations if we optimize bone health throughout life. This can be accomplished with changes in lifestyle that improve not only bone but other important health parameters as well.

Proper Diet

Americans, especially women, are manic about their diet. They combine foods, count calories, manipulate nutrients, buy diet books, deprive themselves, and pay outrageous prices for pills and potions hoping that the "right" diet will bring them the slim look and/or healthy body they crave. This penchant for dieting can have detrimental effects on bone, especially if there are other predisposing factors for osteoporosis.

In fact, the solution to dieting is simple. Instead of focusing on diet for weight loss, begin thinking of diet in the context provided in most dictionaries: a way of choosing foods. Join the mainstream and eat "naturally." Choose a calorie sufficient diet that is lower in fat, lower in sugar (especially added sugar), higher in fiber, balanced, and varied. If you eat a diet that meets dietary guidelines for the milk group, you will get nutrients that can prevent osteoporosis. A calcium supplement should be added for insurance. (See Chapter 13.) In the same way a good foundation in a building sets the stage for the structure over it, a good diet is the foundation for health if you plan to live a long time.

There is growing evidence of a positive link between fruit and vegetable intake and bone health. Fruits and vegetables are rich in potassium, magnesium, beta-carotene, fiber, and vitamin D—dietary elements that facilitate the environment in which bones thrive.

Dietary Calcium

It is so important, we will say it again. A diet low in calcium, at any age, is a shortcut to unhealthy bones. Calcium is the most abundant mineral in the body. About 99 percent of it is stored in your bones. It makes up three pounds of normal body weight. It does more than support the growth of healthy bones. It is also essential for blood clotting, nerve transmission, and muscle contraction. In short, the importance of calcium begins at birth and continues throughout life. Think about it. When we attempt to feed starving children, the first line of defense is often high in protein and calcium powdered milk. Without milk in the formative years bones can't reach maximum density. Adding a high calcium diet later in life can improve bone mineral content and slow bone loss, but by then it is too late to prevent osteoporosis.

Despite what vitamin salespeople tell you, the best-absorbed source of calcium comes from milk and milk products. If you choose low-fat or nonfat milk you get the added benefit of a diet that is lower in fat.

Which Milk Will You Choose?

MILK	Calories/ 8 oz.	mg of CA* /8 oz.	gm. fat/8 oz.
whole milk	150	~ 300	8
2 percent	121	~ 300	4
1 percent	102	~ 300	2
skim	80	~ 325	0

*CA is the abbreviation for calcium
NOTE: Some stores carry calcium fortified milk.

About Milk-Free Diets

People who are proponents of a milk-free diet (what will their bones be like when they are old?) make logical sounding but ridiculous statements including, "Humans are the only species that continue to drink milk after they are weaned." Humans are also the only "species" that get osteoporosis. You will also hear, "Dark green leafy vegetables are excellent sources of calcium." Once again that is only part of the story. Calcium is not as well absorbed from these foods as it is from milk or milk products. Remember, the vitamin D in milk products, which makes calcium more absorbable, isn't present in vegetables. Most of these "you don't need milk" proponents neglect to add that it takes 1 1/2 cups of kale, 3 cups of broccoli, or 10 cups of cabbage to get the amount of calcium found in one glass of milk, 2/3 cup of yogurt, or 1/2 cup of cottage cheese. If you can eat five cups of greens a day, go for it.

We are such strong advocates for milk in the diet you may think we work for the Dairy Council. We don't, but we prefer the milk mustache route.

If you are premenopausal, you need at least 1000 mg of calcium a day.

If you are postmenopausal, you need at least 1200-1500 mg of calcium a day.

Lactose Intolerance

Some people develop intolerance to the milk sugar, lactose, when they get older. Their bodies no longer produce lactase, the enzyme that breaks milk sugar down to glucose. The undigested lactose is eaten in the intestine by bacteria that live there naturally. The gassy waste products produced by the bacteria processing the lactose can create uncomfortable abdominal cramping. If you are lactose intolerant, you may still be able to eat calcium-containing milk products including yogurt, buttermilk, or sour cream. (There are naturally occurring bacteria in these products that break lactose apart.) There is also an over-the-counter product, Lactaid®, which

Eat the following and you will get 300 mg of calcium:

Milk
1/2 cup powdered milk
1 cup milk (skim, 1%, 2%, whole)

Cheese
1 1/2 oz. cheddar-type cheese
2 1/2 oz. American (processed) cheese
1 3/4 oz. mozzarella (part skim milk) cheese

Other Dairy Products
6 oz. low-fat plain yogurt
1 cup low-fat fruited yogurt
1 cup pudding made with milk
1 3/4 cups ice-cream or ice milk

Fish
5 oz. salmon, with bone
7 sardines, with bone

Vegetables
2 cups spinach
2 cups collard greens
3 cups broccoli
10 cups raw cabbage

Calcium fortified foods include:

bread	orange juice
cranberry juice	ready-to-eat cereals
milk	

does what a lactase deficient digestive system cannot. If neither of these strategies work, get a referral from your doctor to meet with a dietitian. That is the best place to get guidelines for managing the calcium (and riboflavin, vitamin D, and protein) deficient diet that occurs when you can't drink milk.

Since we know calcium is important, we also need forewarning about calcium-robbing nutrients in our diet.

Caffeine in Your Diet

The jury is still out. Does or doesn't caffeine increase bone loss? Our research for this book revealed there is no consensus on this question because the "scientific literature" is conflicting. Recent data don't support the long held belief that caffeine is bad for you. If you have been diagnosed with thin bones, take the high road. Don't wait for the scientists to come to a clear conclusion. Caffeine is an addictive drug. Those of us who start our day with a race to the local coffee merchant for a 'latte,' or our neighborhood market for a caffeine-filled Diet Coke®, know it gives our morning a jump-start. The best case scenario, especially when you've been told you have fragile bones, is to limit intake to a couple of cups (or cans) a day. Don't try to remove caffeine from your diet without a slow withdrawal period, or you will have a throbbing headache you will remember for a long time.

Alcohol in Your Diet

Alcohol has been shown to increase the excretion of calcium. Oh yes, we know "a glass or two of red wine a day is good for heart health." But, more than two glasses a day may be too much if you have osteoporosis. Consider limiting yourself to a drink or two a week or as a treat for special occasions.

What You Need to Know:

You are receiving plenty of encouragement from many professionals to maintain a healthy weight. The bottom line, if you will excuse the pun, is that an appropriate diet for someone who has or could get osteoporosis doesn't come with some of the typical "lose weight" dietary advice media perpetuates. Writers and reporters are savvy about your desire to learn how to improve your health. That's why there are so many health-oriented, attention-getting headlines. Some of them are misleading. Remember the Y2K crisis? Nothing came of it. When you hear or read about diet strategies for quick weight loss, think long-term. If healthy eating (and exercise) in your younger years can prevent most diseases of longevity, why not take out an insurance policy now? Instead of eating for results that will make you look good at your high school reunion, or that wedding, or a trip to the beach, begin today to eat for your life.

Chapter Thirteen

Supplements

"I will start taking calcium again."
Judy, Age 53 and many more

Finally, we get to supplements. Two of our most frequently asked questions are, "What should I take?" and "What is the correct dosage?" Thanks to ads, informercials, famous personalities, and neighbors telling you to take this or take that, especially if they are selling this high-profit item, consumers remain confused.

The supplement market, which exploded when shrewd entrepreneurs scurried to take advantage of sloppy 1994 legislation, can bewilder the most savvy health professionals. Suddenly, labels for vitamin, mineral, herbal, hormone, and amino acid products promise cures for and relief from every symptom imaginable. Supplements are sold without the FDA approval that regulates prescription drugs. The Federal Trade Commission (FTC) stepped in with guidelines to assure advertising stays truthful and substantiated, but only a few players in the industry are abiding by those rules.

A Hungry Body

Your body craves many vitamins and minerals every day. These "micronutrients" don't have calories, but without them, you can't digest, absorb, or metabolize the calories you eat. Vitamins and minerals help your body heal injuries, fight disease, and drive the thousands of chemical reactions taking place in your body every second. If you are like most Americans, you are whipping out your wallet and jumping on the supplement bandwagon in an effort to improve your health. Some of you may be carrying a good thing too far by taking many different supplements every day. It's not necessary.

Some of the most exciting developments in the field of nutrition are the new discoveries that identify previously unknown, essential to life, substances in food. With each discovery, a new group of pills is sure to be produced as entrepreneurs take their piece of the vitamin pie. Remember our first rule of thumb: Supplements are not a substitute for food. You are better off using the dietary recommendations in Chapter 12. Go for balance, variety, less sugar, less fat, sufficient calories, and more fiber. Think food first, then supplementation.

Don't get us wrong. We are strong proponents of supplementation in general—especially for calcium and vitamin D that can prevent osteoporosis. But don't go overboard.

Calcium

Whether you are 5, 25, 55, or 85 years young, the amount of calcium in your diet affects the density and strength of your bones now and in the future. Calcium is the most abundant mineral in your body and ninety-nine percent of it is stored in your bones. But it's the "non-bone" functions of calcium that are critical to your bone's ability to retain stored calcium. Muscle contraction, blood clotting, the body's self-defense mechanism to fight infection, even calcium's role in every living cell, all compete for dietary calcium on a daily basis.

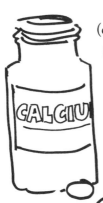

Milk, milk products, fish with bones (canned sardine and canned salmon), and green leafy vegetables are the primary, and best, sources of dietary calcium. If you eat enough of these foods, you will meet your calcium needs. Since many women don't, insurance, in the form of a calcium supplement, is wise.

So which calcium supplement is best? First of all, beware of the word "natural." Calcium is often sold in the form of dolomite, bone meal, or crushed oyster shells because it is "natural." Market experts remind supplement entrepreneurs that if they put the word "natural" in front of the product, their customers will pay up to three times more for them than the identical product without the "natural" moniker. Germs are natural. Disease is natural. Bee stings are natural. Snake bites are natural. We don't want them and neither do you. Natural may be the most overused word in the health promotion field today. Some of these calcium sources are filled with lead or other toxic materials. How's that for natural?

Instead, use a laboratory-produced calcium. There are several. Calcium carbonate is the most popular because it is so inexpensive and it is concentrated; you need only two or three tablets to meet recommended daily allowances for calcium of 1200–1500 milligrams/day. Since many antacids contain calcium carbonate they are often recommended for calcium supplementation. But beware: If the antacid also contains aluminum, the calcium will not be absorbed.

Tums® is the best known of the inexpensive, non-aluminum, non-magnesium, and calcium carbonate containing antacids. It is used as an antacid AND a calcium supplement. Each Tums® contains about 200 mg of elemental calcium. **Remember: your antacid (used for calcium supplementation) should not be taken with food.**

Calcium lactate (lactose = milk sugar) is the best absorbed supplement, but you need to take more calcium lactate because the percentage of elemental calcium (the amount extracted) that can be extracted from this compound is considerably lower than other calcium supplements. The same is true of other calcium supplements, including calcium citrate and calcium gluconate. Calcium must dissolve in your stomach to be absorbed. If your calcium tablet does not dissolve within 30 minutes, it will not be properly absorbed in your body. (The science experiment in Chapter 9 will help you discover how quickly your calcium supplement dissolves.)

The human body absorbs calcium most efficiently in amounts of 500 milligrams per dose or less. Absorption is always enhanced by taking your supplement with meals. You may hear that you should not take your calcium with meals if you eat a high in fiber diet because the fiber can reduce absorption. But all fibers are not alike. Fiber found in grainy foods like oatmeal, fresh fruits, and most vegetables may indirectly help absorb calcium. The only foods that will interfere with the absorption of calcium are beans and foods high in oxalates, like spinach.

You can save money by purchasing 1000 mg tablets and breaking them in two (vs. buying 500-milligram tablets and taking a couple each day). **You can encourage absorption by drinking lots of water between meals.**

Don't be confused by the labels on calcium products that may show the calcium compound and the amount of elemental calcium provided. You are interested in the latter number only. That's how much calcium you will actually receive

Calcium Compound	Elemental Calcium Provided
Calcium Carbonate	40%
Calcium Citrate	21%
Calcium Lactate	13%
Calcium Gluconate	9%

Remember, calcium supplements can't cure osteoporosis. They support bone building and help prevent calcium removal from the bones. We agree with the recommended dietary intake of 1200-1500 milligrams of calcium a day. We prefer you get it from food, but taking 1000 milligrams/day in a calcium supplement, in two divided doses of 500 mg each is the best case scenario. Never take more than 2500 mg of calcium a day. High doses increase the likelihood of developing kidney stones.

Most importantly, to benefit from supplementation, choose a brand made by a reputable company and don't skip your daily dose.

Sunshine and Vitamin D

Want to be sure you get the best absorption and use of calcium? Be sure you get enough vitamin D. Your body cannot absorb calcium from your intestine or make new bone without vitamin D. That doesn't mean you have to take vitamin D with calcium, but it does need to be available from some source.

You receive the vitamin D you need every day in two ways. The ultraviolet rays of the sun on your skin triggers the production of vitamin D by the body. It takes about 15 minutes of exposure every day for your skin to make the vitamin D your body needs. You also get vitamin D in your diet. The best source is fortified milk (yogurt, cottage cheese, and other milk products are NOT fortified with vitamin D). It is also available in some fortified breakfast cereals, and the higher in fat sources, egg yolks and liver.

If you wear sunscreen (which protects you from skin cancer) your body will not get the ultraviolet rays necessary to make vitamin D. Of course, if you become housebound you will not be exposed to the sun. We also know the body's ability to make vitamin D declines with age. That is when vitamin D supplements become a useful adjunct to your diet. Many multi-vitamin/mineral supplements have all the vitamin D you need, and some calcium products are packaged with vitamin D.

Like other fat-soluble vitamins (vitamin E, vitamin K, and vitamin A), vitamin D is measured in international units or IU. We agree with dietary recommendations of 400 IU per day unless you are at risk. In that case it is okay to double the dose to 800 IU per day.

Drink your milk and play outside, especially when it's sunny. After 15 minutes, be sure to put on your sunscreen. Take a general multi-vitamin/mineral product every day and a calcium and vitamin D supplement, and all your bases should be covered.

Other Vitamins and Minerals

Our bones contain many minerals in addition to calcium. Vitamin D, zinc, copper, manganese, boron, magnesium, and vitamin K all play a role in bone health. Calcium and other vitamins and minerals also play a role in many other functions of the body besides bone health. As research about vitamins and minerals continues to evolve, it is certain we will learn about other micronutrients and the role they play in the prevention and treatment of osteoporosis. For today, think diet first, then supplements. If you don't use dairy products, you can take care of your calcium needs with a general multi-vitamin/mineral tablet and calcium supplement. If you want to take a stress vitamin (vitamin Bs) and/or an antioxidant (vitamin C, vitamin E, and zinc), it won't hurt you. If you break the pharmacist Ronda's "rule of five," (taking more than five products each day), you are in overkill and should check with your pharmacist about possible interactions.

Start smart with smart eating.
Supplement with calcium and vitamin D.
Remember the "rule of five." Take no more than five pills a day unless you discuss it with your doctor first!

What You Need to Know:

Supplements can play a vital role in assuring you get nutrients missing in your diet because of chronic illness, dieting, stress, or poor eating habits. Supplements can also pump up the vitamin-mineral content of a decent diet, especially if taken with food in a form that assures they will be well absorbed.

Calcium, the most abundant mineral in the body, cannot cure osteoporosis. However, maintaining adequate blood levels with a calcium-rich diet and calcium supplements can assure bone calcium is not compromised when the body is challenged by other needs for calcium. It is best absorbed in the inexpensive form of calcium carbonate, in doses of 500 mg or less, taken several times a day. Check supplement bottles for the amount of elemental calcium the supplement truly delivers.

Vitamin D plays an important role in the absorption of calcium. Fifteen minutes of exposure to the sun every day can trigger your body to produce the vitamin D you need. Supplementation in the form of fortified foods or the small amount available in a multiple vitamin/mineral tablet can provide useful insurance, especially for people who live in gray winter climates, who use sunscreens, or are who are bedridden. Most calcium supplements come with vitamin D added.

Chapter Fourteen

Exercise: One More Time For Good Measure

"I will begin an exercise program."

Kaye, Age 40

Each fall when trees lose their leaves, homeowners face the awesome task of raking leaves. If, one weekend, they tackle the job, repetitive raking can produce painful blisters that eventually heal, leaving no telltale signs of the effort. But suppose the leaves on the tree fell all year long and our homeowner faced a little bit of leaf raking every day. Instead of blisters you would see calluses.

When you exercise, a similar effect happens to your bones. The repetitive "strike force" or impact of your foot, bearing the weight of your body on a hard surface, reminds your bones to get thicker and harder, so they will be less prone to injury when stressed. It's this impact that is important. Non-impact exercise on bicycles, elliptical exercise machines, or in water are not the best choice for osteoporosis prevention and treatment. The force of pushing a pedal or pulling your arm through water will make you fit and cause some increase in bone density, but it doesn't harden bone as effectively as true impact activities such as walking, jogging, playing tennis, stair climbing, step aerobics, and dancing. However, if balance is an issue, swimming is a wonderful choice and far better than doing nothing at all.

Magnitude of Force + Frequency of Application
creates
Mechanical Stress
and
Electrical Energy
that
Stimulates the Bone
and
Increases the Calcium Content of Bone
resulting in
Bone Hypertrophy (thicker bones)

A bone gets strong in direct proportion to the strength of the muscles attached to it. If you put a rubber band on the end of a stick and pull, you must stabilize the stick to keep it from bending or snapping. If you have a thick stick, you can be less concerned about breakage. The beauty of the relationship between muscle and bone is that when muscles get stronger, bones do too. That's why, in addition to high or low-impact aerobic exercise, doctors are now encouraging women to add upper and lower-body strength training to their fitness routine. Exercise that strengthens the quadricep (front of the thigh) muscles can also improve balance that is lost as we age. Improvement in core muscle strength in the abdominal and pelvic region contribute to better posture and a stable standing and walking stance. A strength-training program can reverse the ravages of inactivity within months. Where else could you get such a terrific return on your investment of time and energy?

Since the accidents that result in broken bones are usually due to a fall, exercises that improve balance, coordination, and flexibility are also important. Learning to balance won't burn a lot of calories or strengthen bones, but the contribution to stability, plus a feeling of well being, and ease in completing daily chores, make balance exercises important for preventing and treating this disease.

If you aren't a fitness buff, it's not too late to start something. Whether you are young or not so young, you'll experience gains. Because exercise cannot be stored, the axiom, "Use it or lose it," applies here. These benefits are short-lived if the program is not continued.

Many people believe that weight bearing exercise means lifting weights. It is not. Weight bearing exercise is exercise done on your feet.

Where Should I Begin?

We agree with the U. S. Surgeon General's report that tells us lack of exercise is dangerous to our health. If you aren't exercising, begin now. If you have a history of health problems or parents with health problems, it's probably wise to check with a physician before you begin this new way of life. You can start with the progressive walking program outlined in the appendix of this book, or use one of many books and videos recommended there to provide the conditioning and strength training that can prevent bone loss and improve bone health.

. . . .

If you have been exercising but your program has been non-weight bearing, or you do only one kind of exercise, consider broadening your perspective. Cross-training (the use of several kinds of exercise), interval training (mixing hard and gentle intensity), strength training, and movement that encourages balance, coordination, and flexibility can take you to a higher level of systemic (including bone) health.

What You Need to Know:

Exercise for prevention and treatment of osteoporosis includes more than the physical effort we usually associate with getting fit. It encompasses all the elements of a total fitness program: systemic aerobic exercise, strength training, balance, coordination, and flexibility. All of these, especially when done on your feet, provide a safe and potent stimulus to maintain and increase bone mass in adults of any age. It's never too early to begin storing bone, and it's never too late to maintain, or even restore bone.

> **The bones of people
> who do impact exercise regularly
> are harder than
> the bones of people
> who do non-impact exercise regularly,
> which are harder than
> the bones of people
> who do no exercise at all.**

Chapter Fifteen

Healthy Lifestyle

"Great reinforcement for avoiding cigarettes"

Amy, Age 28

We've covered all the dietary and lifestyle issues we know are important to prevent osteoporosis except two, smoking and stress reduction.

Smoking — Again

As little as ten years ago smoking was cool. There were ashtrays on restaurant tables and circular sand-filled bins in front of elevator doors in department stores. "Back then" you could even smoke in an airplane. Then a shift began. We both remember the early days of that shift. Friends and relatives with the cigarette habit criticized Ronda for posting and enforcing a "no smoking" sign at her home. Beverly remembers visits by her mother who stood in front of the Whipple home, cigarette in hand, complaining to every passing neighbor about her "mean daughter" who wouldn't let her smoke in the house.

My, how times have changed! Tobacco companies admit they added addiction-producing nicotine to cigarettes. Many states have declared public places must be smoke free. Although there are still mini ashtrays on the arms of airplane seats and in their lavatories, if you light up you will set off alarms and be evicted at the next stop. (Some people believe smokers should be evicted mid-flight!) People who smoke at work must do it outside the building. Smoking kills. Smoke one pack of cigarettes a day for 20 years and it's almost certain you will get lung cancer.

In Chapter 5 you learned smoking is a potent risk factor for osteoporosis. Nicotine increases estrogen breakdown and decreases the population of osteoblasts that build bones. If you smoke, you are more likely to go through menopause earlier, depriving your body of a few additional years of bone-strengthening estrogen protection.

If you smoke, stop. We agree it's easier said than done, but there are excellent programs and products to support withdrawal. **If you don't smoke, don't start. It isn't cool. It's deadly.** (See the appendix for stop smoking resources.)

Stress Reduction

Your emotional outlook and attitude can impact how you deal with the lifestyle changes that prevent and/or treat osteoporosis. The key is taking care of yourself.

Set aside time each day (even if it is just a few minutes) for relaxation. Attempt to release negative feelings. Mentally, give your stress away or, symbolically, put it in something you can destroy. The emerging research about the physiological and psychological benefits gained by brief breaks, reflective time, mental exercise, and recreation can't be denied.

Consider the use of positive affirmations to support new

bone-building habits. At first, the use of this behavior-changing tool may feel uncomfortable. "How can I affirm what isn't true?" "This feels awkward," or "I think this is stupid," are just a few of the comments we hear when we make this suggestion.

Use these guidelines to get started:

- Begin your affirmation with the word, "I." This is a strong statement of your personal power.
- Always affirm in the now. Instead of saying, "My bones are getting stronger," say, "My bones are stronger."
- Omit the word "should" from affirmations. It's a dangerous word anytime. Instead of "I should...," say, "I do."
- Avoid using the words "no," "non," "not," and "never." "I no longer fall down," or "I never fall," are powerful reminders you are changed, but they are negative. A more useful choice is "I am poised and confident and have steady feet." "I have excellent balance."
- Avoid using the words "hope," wish," and "try." They are vague and suggest the possibility of failure. Have you ever "tried" to pick up your car keys? You reach out and pick them up! It is much easier, it takes less energy to do things than to "try to" or "want to" or "need to" do them. Instead of "I am trying to exercise every day," or "I want to exercise every day," affirm, "I exercise daily." (Of course you have to put some effort with the affirmation.)
- Don't slip into self-abusive speaking patterns. Whenever you catch yourself using this language add the phrase "up until now." It reverses the self-defeating message about to be stored in your brain. "I always forget to take my calcium supplement," becomes, "I always forget to take my calcium supplement, up until now."

After you create your affirmation, repeat it to yourself

several times. If it feels somewhat comfortable you have chosen well. Most people need to adjust the wording of their affirmation until it seems "right."

Here are some affirmations that have worked for women like yourself:

"I care about myself and my body."

"Every day I do what is necessary to be healthy."

"I exercise, eat smart, and take my calcium to prevent osteoporosis."

"I stand straight and tall. I have no fractures."

What You Need to Know:

A healthy lifestyle is a smoke-free lifestyle. It includes strategies to manage stress, a positive attitude, and a consistent effort to affirm and practice habits that say, "I care about me."

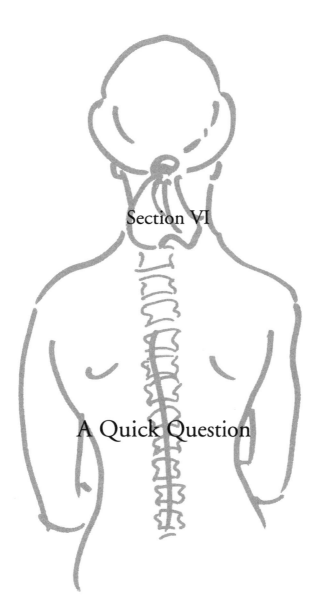

Section VI

A Quick Question

"I got all my questions answered"
Paula, Age 44

Chapter Sixteen

A Quick Question

"Thanks for answering my questions about osteoporosis."
Ethel, age 52

It always makes us smile when someone approaches us after a lecture and says, "I have a quick question." Quick questions rarely require quick answers. Since many are repeated often, we've included some of them here hoping one will apply to your specific problem.

I'm 45 years old. When do I need to start worrying about the health of my bones?

Women should be concerned about their bones their entire life. The diet and exercise patterns of adolescence determine the maximum density of bones up to age 30 or so. After that, serious bone loss occurs silently, years before the damage is evident. That includes a loss of about 1 percent a year beginning in your mid-thirties. In the five to seven years following menopause, women can lose up to 20 percent of bone mass without knowing it. See Chapter 3 to assess your own risk and Chapters 12, 13, 14, and 15 to learn more about the lifestyle that can prevent poor bone health.

I just had a DEXA scan, which was normal. Am I safe?

The DEXA test measures your bone density at the moment but tells you nothing about any ongoing rate of bone loss. You need to be tested at least every two years with another DEXA scan to discover if your lifestyle is maintaining bone mass. See Chapters 12, 13, 14, and 15.

Is it true that when I get old I will be frail and weak and there is nothing I can do about it?

You have almost everything to do with the quality of your life in the future. Weakness, stooped shoulders, broken hips, shoulders, and wrists can be avoided with a combination of exercise, a nutritionally adequate diet, proper supplementation and, for many women, estrogen replacement therapy. See Chapters 12, 13, 14, and 15.

Is it true that once I have lost bone, it is gone forever?

No. If bone loss is detected early enough, proper medication and changes in lifestyle can encourage the growth of new bone.

How can I help my children and grandchildren prevent osteoporosis?

Teach your daughters and grandchildren that most of the diseases of aging, including osteoporosis, don't happen overnight. Remind them that most disease progresses silently until there is a crisis that reveals the results of poor lifestyle choices at an earlier age. This is particularly true with osteoporosis. Encourage them to drink milk instead of juice or soda pop, eat a healthy diet, avoid dieting, smoking, and excessive use of alcohol. Provide smart guidance about the supplements they can use to synergize the good lifestyle habits that can build and maintain bone and prevent osteoporosis (and other diseases of aging). And, as you teach, practice what you preach.

Won't I gain weight on a calcium-rich diet?

Smart eating includes the use of high-in-calcium dairy products that are also low in fat and sugar. You can get the same amount of calcium in a serving of skim milk (80 calories) that you can get with a serving of whole milk (156 calories). The same is true for other skim and low fat milk based products including the cheese, yogurt, and low fat frozen desserts you and your family can enjoy without worrying about gaining weight. Of course, you must exercise and be sure that you don't eat more calories than you burn. That's what weight management is about—balancing the intake and output of calories.

How do I know which drug is right for me?

You and your health-care provider are partners in determining what medications are right for you. This is based on your health history, your risk factors, and the results of your DEXA scan.

How much calcium do my children and I need?

The National Institutes of Health's Developmental Conference on Optimal Calcium Intake makes the following recommendations:

Ages 1-3:   500 mg/day
Ages 4-8:   800 mg/day
Ages 9-18:   1,300 mg/day
Age 19-50:   Prior to menopause: 1000 mg/day
                Premature menopause 1500 mg/day
Age 50-65:   After menopause with estrogen therapy:
                1000-1200 mg/day
                After menopause without estrogen therapy:
                1500 mg/day
Over Age 65:   1500 mg/day

How much calcium does my infant need?

Infants from birth to six months need 210 mg of calcium a day, and infants from six months to one year need 270 mg a day.

Do I need more calcium when I am pregnant or breast-feeding?

Pregnant and lactating women need to add 400mg/day to the above doses.

Is it possible to take too much calcium?

Most experts are not worried about the risk of excessive inake but also recommend you don't routinely exceed 2500 milligrams a day. For the best absorption, space your calcium intake throughout the day.

I can't exercise. What can I do to help prevent osteo-porosis?

Sorry. We don't buy into the "can't exercise" excuse. Unless you can't move there is always something you can do. Work with a sports medicine physician or physical therapist to find a way to overcome your barriers. This is especially important for women who have weak muscles. See Chapter 14.

My elderly mother was diagnosed with osteoporosis. She's on medication and sees a physical therapist. Do you have any other suggestions to support her care?

Since falls are so dangerous for people who have osteoporosis, here are some tips that can make your mother's living environment safer.
- Be sure all carpets, especially area rugs, have skid-proof backings.
- If a floor is waxed, it is slippery. Give up the shine.

- Install grab bars in the bathroom to make sitting down, standing up, and moving in and out of a tub or shower safer.
- Spend time with your mother so you can identify which items she uses frequently. Then put them within easy reach. This includes pens, pencils, notepads, soap and toilet paper in the bathroom, and food in the refrigerator.
- If your mother is unsteady, buy her a cane or walker to support her confidence to keep moving.

I have three small children. I am almost always carrying one of them. Is that enough weight bearing exercise?

Carrying children is good weight bearing exercise, but it is not enough to prevent osteoporosis because you are doing only one kind of lifting. To prevent osteoporosis you need to strengthen your upper body muscles in several ways. The books listed on page 154 will give you all the information you need.

Also be sure you understand that weight bearing describes two different kinds of exercise. In addition to the strength training suggested above, it is important to move your feet.

Experts often argue about which is best for bones. Instead of choosing one, do both. Strength (or resistance) train *and* get into a physical activity program that requires your foot to strike a hard surface. Walking, jogging, stepping, kick boxing and dancing are just a few of the options that work well when you want to build and maintain bone. (See Ronda's Smart Walking program on page 157.)

Glossary

Actonel®: Trade name for risedronate, a bisphosphonate approved for the prevention and treatment of post-menopausal osteoporosis produced by Procter & Gamble Pharmaceuticals and Aventis Pharmaceuticals.

Aerobic: Literally means "with oxygen."

Aerobic Exercise: Exercise that requires oxygen in the muscle to process stored body fat for muscle work. For the purpose of osteoporosis prevention and treatment this includes walking, jogging, dancing, stair climbing, and other exercise done on the feet on a hard surface.

Alendronate: generic name for the bisphosphonate, Fosamax®. (See Fosamax®)

Amenorrhea: A lack of menstrual periods.

Anaerobic: Literally means "without oxygen."

Anaerobic Exercise: Exercise that does not require oxygen in the muscle to process energy for muscle work. Strength training, done with weights or elastic bands, is an excellent anaerobic exercise strategy to maintain and build dense bones. It also increases metabolism.

Bisphosphonates: A group of drugs that have the ability to attach to calcium in bone and prevent osteoclasts from breaking down the bone.

Bone Density: Describes the amount of calcium and mineral in bone.

Bone mineral density (BMD): BMD is the abbreviation for Bone Mineral Density. BMD testing measures the density of bones in men and women of all ages.

Calcimar®: Trade name for salmon calcitonin, an injection approved by FDA for post-menopausal treatment of osteoporosis; produced by Rhone-Poulene Rorer.

Calcitonin: A hormone produced in the thyroid gland that takes part in the regulation of calcium metabolism.

Calcium: The most important mineral in bone. Calcium plays an essential role in development and maintenance of a healthy skeleton. If intake is inadequate, calcium is mobilized from the skeleton to maintain normal blood calcium level.

Calcium carbonate: A naturally occurring form of calcium commonly used in calcium supplements.

Calcium citrate: A man made form of calcium used in calcium supplements.

Compression fracture: A collapsed fracture of a vertebra or bone in the spine.

Cortical bone: The dense (hard) outer layer of bone.

Corticosteroid: a group of hormonal substances produced in the adrenal gland. The term is also used to describe a group of medicines that duplicate these substances. Cortisone and prednisone are two well known versions of these drugs.

Dual-energy x-ray absorptiometry (DXA or DEXA): A diagnostic test used to assess bone density in the spine, hip, or wrist using radiation exposure about one tenth that of a standard chest x-ray.

ERT: The abbreviation for estrogen replacement therapy. ERT is prescribed for women who have had a hysterectomy.

Estrace®: An oral estrogen, manufactured by Bristol-Myers Squibb, approved by the FDA for the prevention of osteoporosis

Estraderm®: Trade name for 17 beta-estradiol patch approved by the FDA for the prevention of osteoporosis; produced by Novartis Pharmaceuticals.

Estratab®: Trade name for esterified estrogen, approved by the FDA for the prevention of osteoporosis; produced by Solvay Pharmaceuticals.

Estrogen: One of a group of steroid hormones that control female sexual development.

Estrogen Replacement Therapy: Estrogen replacement therapy. This is prescribed for women who have had a hysterectomy.

Exercise: An intervention long associated with strong bones. This includes aerobic exercise done on a hard surface and strength training anaerobic exercise. Coordination, balance, and flexibility exercises improve balance and can prevent falls.

. . . .

Evista®: Trade name for raloxifene, a selective estrogen receptor modulator (SERM) approved by the FDA for the prevention and treatment of osteoporosis; produced by Eli Lilly & Co.

Family history: A risk factor for osteoporosis fractures; defined as a maternal and/or paternal history of hip, wrist, or spine fracture when the parent was age 50 years or older.

Fluoride: A compound that stimulates the formation of new bone by enhancing the recruitment and differentiation of osteoblasts.

Fosamax®: Trade name for alendronate, a bisphosphonate approved by the FDA for the for prevention and treatment of osteoporosis; produced by Merck & Co.

Fracture: A break in a bone.

Hormone replacement therapy (HRT): A general term for all types of estrogen replacement therapy (ERT) when given along with progesterone, either cyclically or continuously. HRT is generally prescribed for women after natural menopause or surgical removal of both ovaries.

HRT: the abbreviation for hormone replacement therapy.

Low bone mass: See osteopenia.

Menopause: The completion of the ovarian transition, marked by the last menstrual period (menopause is considered complete when a woman has been without menstrual periods for one year).

Miacalcin®: Trade name for salmon calcitonin, a nasal spray approved by FDA for post-menopausal treatment of osteoporosis; produced by Sandoz Pharmaceuticals.

Normal bone mass: The designation for bone density within 1 standard deviation of the mean for young normal adults (T-score above –1).

Ogen®: Trade name for piperazine estrone sulfate, approved by FDA for the prevention of osteoporosis; produced by Upjohn.

Ossification: The process by which cartilage is converted to hard bone.

Osteoblast: A cell that forms bone.

Osteoclast: A cell that breaks down bone.

Osteopenia: A condition characterized by a decrease in bone density that makes it too low to be normal, but not low enough to render a diagnosis of osteoporosis. (T-scores between –1 and –2.5).

Osteoporosis: A chronic, progressive disease characterized by low bone mass and deterioration of bone tissue, leading to bone fragility and an increase in risk of fracture (T-scores at or below –2.5).

Peak bone mass: The maximum bone mass achieved during skeletal growth. It occurs at young adulthood.

Peripheral fractures: Nonvertebral or non-spine fractures including, those of the hip, wrist, forearm, leg, ankle, foot, rib, sternum, and other sites.

Premarin®: Trade name for conjugated estrogen, an oral estrogen replacement therapy approved by the FDA for the prevention and management of osteoporosis, produced by Wyeth Ayerst. (Premarin® = made from pregnant mares urine).

Prevention of osteoporosis: The practice of preventing bone mineral density from dropping lower than 2.5 standard deviations below the mean for young normal adult women; commonly used to describe the prevention of osteoporosis-related fractures.

Previous fracture: A risk factor for fractures; defined here as a history of a previous fracture after age 40.

Raloxifene: generic name for the SERM, Evista®; see Evista®.

Remodeling: An ongoing dual process of bone formation (by osteoblasts) and bone resorption (by osteoclasts) in an adult.

Resistance training: (also known as strength training): A method of strengthening muscle by increasing the force of contraction of the muscle by using weights, elastic bands, or other strategies. This effort, performed consistently, creates a force on bone that increases its density.

Resorption: The loss of substance (in this case bone) through physiological or pathological means.

Risedronate: generic name for the new bisphosphonate, Actonel®; See Actonel®.

Risk factors: Factors that increase the risk of something happening. Osteoporosis risk factors include: low bone mineral density, a genetic predisposition to the disease, excessively low body weight or small frame size, previous fracture, a sedentary lifestyle, and smoking.

Single x-ray absorptiometry (SXA): A diagnostic test used to assess bone density. It is NOT used to measure bone density in the hip or spine but is useful for peripheral sites.

Steroids: a class of synthesized chemical compounds that mimic hormones. They include estrogen, testosterone, cortisone, and prednisone.

Standard deviation (SD): A measure of variation of a distribution.

Strength Training: See resistance training.

Trabecular bone: the soft, spongy-like inner core of bone

T-score: In describing bone mineral density (BMD), the number of standard deviations above or below the mean for young normal adults.

Ultrasound densitometry: A diagnostic test used to assess bone density at the ankle or knee.

Vitamin D: A fat-soluble vitamin useful to prevent and treat osteoporosis.

Weight Bearing Exercise: Exercise that is done in an upright position, with the feet impacting a hard surface. Some popular weight bearing exercises are walking, running, stair-stepping, stair climbing, skating, dancing, tennis, and gymnastics.

Appendix A

Osteoporosis Risk Factor Profile

To help determine your risk of osteoporosis, circle the number next to the statement in each category that is most true for you. Add up the points when you have finished the entire profile.

Genetic factors

Age:

Under 35	1
35-50	3
51-65	7
Over 65	12

Heritage

African-American	1
Asian	2
Mediterranean or Middle Eastern	3
Caucasian	5

Complexion:

Dark	1
Ruddy/Olive	2
Fair/Pale	3

Family History:

No known bone problems in family	1
Relative over 60 with bone disease	3
Parent with bone disease	4
Relative under 60 with bone disease	5

Wrist size:

Over 6.5"	1
6" - 6.5 "	2
5" – 6"	3
Under 5"	4

Height:

Over 5'8"	1
5'5" – 5'8"	2
5'2" – 5'5"	3
Under 5'2"	4

Body type:

Mesomorphic- high muscle, low fat	1
Endomorphic- high fat, low muscle	6
Ectomorphic- low fat, low muscle	6

Onset of Menopause:

After age 50	1
Age 46-50	3
Age 45 or under*	5
Surgical menopause age 45 or under*	7

* deduct 5 points if estrogen therapy was started within one year after surgery or early menopause. Deduct 3 points if started more than three years after surgery or early menopause.

My Genetic Score _____

Lifestyle Factors

Exercise (total body):
4 or more time a week	0
1-3 times a week	3
At least 3 times a month	6
Avoid physical activity	12

Calcium Intake:
4 or more servings of low-fat dairy products a day	0
More than 2 servings a day	3
2 or less servings a day	6
Avoid dairy products	12

Protein Intake:
Avoid red meat	0
Eat only seafood and white meat poultry	1
Eat meat 3 times a week or less	3
Eat meat 4 times a week or more	6

Caffeine Consumption:
Avoid caffeine and tannin beverages	0
Decaffeinated drinks and/or tea only	2
3 cups or less of coffee/tea daily	3
4 cups or more coffee daily	6

Alcohol Consumption:
Less than
2 beers, 8 oz wine or
3 oz. of spirits per week 0
2-4 beers, 8-16 oz wine or
3-6 oz spirits per week 2
Up to 2 beers, 8 oz wine or
3 oz spirits per day 4
More than 2 beers, 16 oz wine
or 6 oz spirits per day 8

Tobacco Use:
Non smoker 0
Less than 14 cigarettes per week 2
Less than 10 cigarettes per day 5
10 cigarettes or more per day 8

My Lifestyle Score _____

My Genetic Score _____

My Total Score _____

What your score means:
8-25 points: your risk factor is well below average
26-48 points: your risk factor is average
49-82 points: you are at moderate risk for developing
  osteoporosis
83-100 points: you are at considerable risk for developing
  osteoporosis

Author unknown

Appendix B

Osteoporosis Risk Factors

- Menopause
- Early menopause (before age 45)
- Abnormal absence of menstrual periods
- Thin or small frame
- Advanced age
- Family history of osteoporosis
- Excessive use of caffeine
- Anorexia nervosa or bulimia
- Use of tobacco
- Excessive use of alcohol
- Sedentary lifestyle
- Of Caucasian or Asian race (Although African-Americans and Hispanics-Americans are also at risk)
- Chronic use of steroids, excessive thyroid hormone, certain anticonvulsants
- Insufficient milk, especially between ages of one and sixteen
- No pregnancies

Appendix C

Questions to Ask Your Doctor

Speaking with your doctor about osteoporosis will help you better understand your own risk for the disease as well as available prevention or treatment options. Listed below are several questions that are intended to help you discuss osteoporosis with your doctor:

- Based on my medical history, lifestyle, and family background, am I at risk for osteoporosis?

- How do I know if someone in my family suffered from osteoporosis? (What physical signs or symptoms should I be looking for?)

- Am I currently taking any medication that puts me at higher risk for developing osteoporosis?

- How do I best prevent (or treat) osteoporosis?

- How do I know if my bone density is low?

- How much calcium is right for me?

- How do I best obtain this calcium?

- Should I engage in exercise? What kind of exercise is best? How often should I exercise?

- How do I know if I have fractured a bone in my spine?

If you have osteoporosis or if your doctor believes you are at high risk for the disease, you may want to ask the following questions:

- What medications are available to help me?

- What are the benefits/side effects of these medications?

- Will these medications interact with other medications I am already taking for other conditions?

- How do I know that my prevention or treatment program is effective?

- Do any of the medications I am taking for other conditions cause dizziness, light-headedness, disorientation, or a loss of balance that could lead to a fall?

Appendix D

Useful Internet Sites

Speaking of Women's Health
http://www.speakingofwomenshealth.com,
http://www.swh.net

We love this organization. If you have attended a Speaking of Women's Health conference you know why. Each year the non-profit foundation manages conferences in more than twenty cities nationwide for the purpose of educating women to make better informed decisions about their health and well-being. The site lists conference locations, reviews the history of the foundation, reviews presentations by the prestigious speakers at each event, and provides useful health information for use in your daily life. Write to: Speaking of Women's Health Foundation, Kathy DeLaura, Executive Director, 1223 Central Parkway, Cincinnati, OH 45214-2890. Telephone: 513-345-6570

National Osteoporosis Foundation
http://www.nof.org

The National Osteoporosis Foundation, established in 1986, is a voluntary non-profit health organization whose mission is to reduce and ultimately eliminate the widespread prevalence of osteoporosis through programs of research, education, and advocacy. A $25 membership entitles you to a quarterly newsletter, Osteoporosis Report and 70 page handbook, Boning Up on Osteoporosis. Write to: National Osteoporosis Foundation, 1150 17th St. Suite 500, Washington, DC, 20036-4603, Telephone: 202-223-2226, FAX: 202-223-2237

The NOF Chicago office manages _a database of physician's who specialize in osteoporosis_ and _a database that lists support groups nationwide_. If there is no support group in your area, the NOF staff will help you start one.
Telephone: 312-464-5110

The Doctor's Guide to the Internet
http://www.pslgroup.com/OSTEOPOROSIS.HTM
The latest medical news and information for patients or friends/parents of patients diagnosed with osteoporosis and osteoporosis-related disorders.

National Institutes of Health Osteoporosis and Related Bone Diseases National Resource Center
http://www.osteo.org
NIHORBD's mission is to provide patients, health professionals, and the public with important resources and information on metabolic bone diseases, including osteoporosis. Write to: NIHORBD, 1232 22nd Street, NW, Washington, DC 20037-1292,
Telephone Toll-free: 800-624-BONE

North American Menopause Society
http://www.menopause.org
This non-profit membership organization is dedicated to promoting understanding of menopause, and improving the health of women as they approach menopause and beyond. Their information is accurate and unbiased. In addition to useful information on the site itself, they offer membership, which includes a subscription to their newsletter, FLASHES!! (great name!) The North American Menopause Society, P.O. Box 94527, Cleveland, Ohio 44101-4527, Telephone: 440-442-7550

EndrocineWeb.com-The Osteoporosis Center
http://www.endocrineweb.com/osteoporosis
This site is an excellent adjunct to SMART WOMEN, STRONG BONES. Much of the information is the same as that in the book, said in a different way. There are support groups and user forums and an "unofficial" listing of physicians suggested by site users. Internet contact only.

The American Society for Bone and Mineral Research (ASBMR)
http://www.asbmr.org
ASBMR encourages and promotes the study of bone and mineral metabolism through annual scientific meetings, an official journal (Journal of Bone and Mineral Research), the Primer on the Metabolic Bone Diseases and Disorders of Mineral Metabolism, and cooperation with other related societies. Write to: ASBMR, 1200 19th Street, NW, Suite 300, Washington, DC 20036-2422,
Telephone: 202-857-1161

The US National Library of Medicine's MedLine Plus Health Information
http://www.nlm.nih.gov/medlineplus
MEDLINEplus is a gold mine of up-to-date, quality health care information from the world's largest medical library, the National Library of Medicine at the National Institutes of Health. Its experienced staff of information experts reviews hundreds of government and non-government publications, brochures, databases, and Web sites in order to link the public with the most reliable and authoritative information.

ibreast.com
http://www.ibreast.com
Dr. Marisa Weiss, author of <u>Living Beyond Breast Cancer</u>, has created a web site that helps women make informed decisions about breast cancer including: prevention, treatment, detection, recovery, diagnosis, and living beyond the disease. It includes a chapter that addresses health issues that includes osteoporosis. Internet contact only.

American Dietetic Association
http://www.eatright.org
Promoting optimal nutrition, health, and well being to consumers through various programs and services is the ADA mission. A consumer nutrition source that includes a referral service to registered dietitians and a resource library with access to an extensive array of databases make ADA a leading source of objective food and nutrition information.

LIFESTYLES by Ronda Gates
Health Promotion Education
http://www.rondagates.com

This site, hosted by *Smart Women, Strong Bones* co-author and Speaking of Women's Health keynoter, Ronda Gates, includes updated information about health issues related to exercise, nutrition, weight control, and stress management. There is a free fitness tip and free recipe daily. Registration for Gates' complimentary weekly Email Newsletter will get you a download of low fat, easy-to-fix recipes. Write to: LIFESTYLES by Ronda Gates, P. O. Box 974, Lake Oswego, OR 97034. Telephone: 503-697-7572

National Dairy Council
http://www.nationaldairycouncil.org

Have you seen the popular milk mustache advertisements produced by this organization? Perhaps you've seen them at health events where they supply the camera and toothpaste concoction so you, too, can sell the "drink milk" message. The national organization provides nutrition information through state, and regional dairy council units. Instead of using this site, use a search engine to search, for "dairy+council" or "dairy + (your state here)" to find your state organization. Write to: National Dairy Board, National Dairy Council, 10255 W. Higgins Rd., Suite 900, Rosemont, IL 60018, Telephone: 312-847-2000

Appendix E

Books and Videos to Support Good Exercise and Eating Habits

Books

The Ultimate Fit or Fat
by Covert Bailey

Covert Bailey's done it again. He's revised his popular Fit or Fat. Though retired from public speaking, as a writer, Bailey remains at the top of his game. The title is misleading. The perspective is based on the necessity to address fitness issues from the perspective of the fit and not so fit. There is a focus in this edition (the 3rd Fit or Fat) on weight lifting–highly recommended by your authors to strengthen the bones of the upper body and jump start your metabolism. The book includes a guide, with pictures, for a home strength bulding program.

Strength Training Past 50
by Wayne L. Westcott, Ph.D, Thomas R. Baechle, Mark Williams

Strength training is an equal-opportunity exercise system. Regardless of how old you are when you start, strength training has nearly immediate benefits: more muscle mass, more strength, a higher fat burning metabolism. This book gives older exercisers all the information they need to get started, including advice on testing for strength and how to pick a qualified personal trainer. Fitness expert Wayne Westcott and supporter Tom Baechle present 39 safe and effective exercises as part of a 10-week strength training plan. 130 photos.

We have a problem with the "for Dummies" books as we don't believe any woman is a dummy. Just close your eyes to get past the title and into the useful information inside the following three books.

Fitness for Dummies
by Suzanne Schlosberg, Liz Neporent

This book is a perfect starter for fitness novices interested in general fitness information. You will learn everything you need to know about starting and maintaining a fitness program—getting motivated, choosing a gym, building strength and aerobic endurance, and buying home exercise equipment. These well-known health writers tell it with wit and style.

Workouts for Dummies
by Tamilee Webb, Lori Seeger

O. K. So you think you can't relate to a buffed star of exercise videos and TV appearances. (Forget your prejudice. Ronda, who knows Tamilee, reports she is the most down-to-earth, enthusiastic motivator you could meet.) This book starts with topics as basic as choosing shoes and warming up. Then it covers everything you'll need to create an effective exercise program, starting with an explanation of body types (so you don't think you'll end up looking like Cindy Crawford if you don't already) and the workouts that suit your body type. The book gives directions for stretches, aerobic exercises, muscle conditioning (using weights, furniture, exercise bands, and bars), and workouts for different locations.

Weight Training for Dummies
by Suzanne Schlosberg, Liz Neporent

If you want a more strenuous strength-training program using free weights and gym machines, try this book, which has plenty of easy-to-understand instructions for beginners, but also includes information for those who've been training a while. It's pumped up with more than 100 photos and illustrations of the best exercises for the major and minor muscle groups—exactly what you need for an osteoporosis-prevention workout.

Smart Eating
by Ronda Gates and Covert Bailey

This book offers an alternative to dieting with a revolutionary way to think about food as nutrition. It uses simple guidelines to let you make the food choices that assure you get the nutrients you need for good osteoporosis prevention and general health (and weight loss). The process is simplified by the Smart Eating "Food Target" — a unique graphic that grades foods according to their fat and fiber content.

Smart Eating is designed for anyone who wants to eat smart—men & women, vegetarians, people with weight problems, athletes, healthy people, and even those with medical problems like osteoporosis and diabetes. It includes 200 recipes keyed to the Food Target. You'll never diet again. Call 1-800-863-6000 or visit Ronda's website: http://www.rondagates.com for a discounted copy plus a free Smart Eating poster.

Nutrition Nuggets
by Ronda Gates

Although this book is ten years old, it is filled with useful information for women of all ages seeking to improve their education about nutrition. In addition to easy-to-read, never out of date text about caffeine, salt, sugar, the various fats, supermarket savvy, and restaurant survival there are ten motivating stories about women who struggled and made lifestyle change. Usually costing $11, the book is available for $5 to readers of this book. Call 1-800-863-6000 or visit Ronda's website: http://www.rondagates.com for a copy.

Home Exercise Videos

http://www.collagevideo.com

This site offers a 60-90 second preview of the several hundred videos they stock. They also have a paper catalog that describes every video available and a toll free service with telephone representatives who can help you choose the video that matches your needs and fitness level. Call 1-800-433-6769 or Email collage@collagevideo.com for a catalog.

http://www.homeworkout.com

There is no catalog for this company and no toll free consultation service but they have a slightly different selection of videos, sell some books and exercise equipment, and offer profiles of exercise leaders.

Smoking Cessation Programs

Ready, Set, Stop

Registered nurse, health educator Fern Carness, a former smoker, has created a 4-tape audio series, program worksheets, food and activity planners, and other materials to help smokers stop their smoking habit.
http://www.readysetstop.com or call: 1-800-950-9355
or write: P. O. Box 509, Lake Oswego, OR 97034

Smokenders

9617 N.W. Golden Avenue, Vancouver, WA 98665, Telephone: 1-800-828-HELP; Web Site: http://www.smok-enders.com. "SMOKENDERS is an educational program having as its goal, not only the cessation of smoking, but of enjoying not smoking and being comfortable as a nonsmoker."

Appendix F

Smart Walking

"The way out is via the door."

-Chinese sage, Lao Tse

When it comes to our country's top exercise, we're voting with our feet. Nearly 22 million Americans walk for fitness at least twice a week. Research shows that walking, which has the lowest drop-out rate of any fitness activity, can make bones stronger AND give you one hour of longevity for every hour you pound the pavement. Start here for a successful fitness program that supports strong bones.

Proper Gear

Shoes:
Athletic shoe companies manufacture shoes designed specifically for walking. Ideally, invest in a pair of walking or cross-training shoes. If your pace gets very fast, running shoes may be more comfortable. Whatever shoes you decide to buy, make sure they have these characteristics:
- A firm, well-cushioned, flexible sole.
- Sturdy uppers made from materials that "breathe."
- Shoes with variable lacing options are best to achieve a custom fit.
- Expect a good walking shoe to support your foot for 3-6 months of daily use then retire them to the garden and invest in another pair.

About the fit:
- Since it's not unusual for your foot to swell by one-half size during the day, buy your shoes as late in the day as possible.

- If, like most people, one of your feet is bigger than the other, choose shoe size based on the larger foot.
- There should be about 1/2 inch between the end of your longest toe and the front of the shoe.
- The toe box of your shoe should be as wide as possible without allowing the heel to slip. Shoe people use words like firm heel counter to describe this feature.
- If you have high-arched feet you'll need cushioning in your shoe to absorb shock when a forcefully propelled foot hits the ground. If you have a low arch (flat feet), your shoe should have greater support and heel control.

Clothes:

If you're walking at a pace sufficient to gain health benefits, you will get hot as you walk. Dress in "layers" that can be removed as needed. In hot weather, dress to permit circulation of air across your skin. If you walk in cold or rainy weather, choose cotton or wool because its "breathability" will absorb sweat without chilling you. Outdoor recreational stores carry exercise gear made from the newer "breathable" fabrics. These garments combine durability, fashion, and the features that keep you warm and dry—essential to a satisfactory experience.

Safety

- If you've never exercised or have a family history of health problems, check with your doctor regarding your suitability to begin an exercise program.
- Always carry some form of identification with you.
- If you walk alone, let someone know where you're going and when you plan to return.
- Never walk alone in parking garages, stairwells, or less populated areas or at night.

- If you'll be walking more than 30 minutes, carry a water bottle. Always carry water on a hot day—even when your walk is short.
- Wear reflective clothing when walking at night.
- Vary your route from day to day.
- If your route is along streets without sidewalks, always face oncoming traffic (unless on a blind bend). Stay as close as possible to the side of the road.
- Follow all traffic signals—always!
- Be aware of activity around you. Keep an eye out for stray dogs, cars, runners, bicyclists, or suspicious characters.
- If you wear a headphone to hear a CD or tape cassette, keep the volume low enough that you can hear what's happening around you. Be EXTRA cautious at intersections.

Smart Walking Technique and Training

Technique

Ronda's mentor, Dr. George Sheehan, fondly known as the running doctor, used to give her a lot of "static" when he heard she led walking classes and taught participants proper walking technique. "Everybody knows how to walk," he said. Then she led him on one of her fitness walks where he was forced to put forth an effort that, for him, was more intensive than his well integrated and efficient running pace. She shared "techniques" for fitness walking to which he responded, "Can you put that down on paper?" This is what she wrote:

"Stand with feet hip width apart. Lift your shoulders, pull them back, then gently press them down. Without losing your ability to breathe deeply, flatten your belly button against your spine as you think about pointing your tail bone toward the ground. Now pull your chin in and lift your head so your eyes are looking forward. Begin to walk, leaning slightly forward from your ankles and bending your arms at your elbows with your palms facing inward. Move your arms in opposition to your feet focusing on the effort that moves your elbows back. As your arm comes forward it should not go above the bustline. Now focus on your foot roll. Heel strike, roll through the foot, and push off with the forefoot and toes."

Training

Smart Walking utilizes Ronda's Smart Heart Rate Training Techniques. Walking pace is divided into three zones that correspond with the metabolic effects generated by the intensity of the zone. These are:

Level One: Health Zone   16-25 minute mile
Level Two: Fitness Zone   12-16 minute mile
Level Three: Performance Zone   <12 minute mile

To determine your current level, you will need to go to a track (4 circuits = 1 mile) or measure, by driving, a one mile distance.

If you can walk that far, record your time for the walk. If you can't make a mile, figure the time for the distance traveled and convert it to a mile. Use the following program e to slowly increase your pace. If you are already fit enough to skip introductory weeks, find the appropriate week that matches your current pace and begin there.

Benefits of Smart Walking

The HEALTH benefits of Smart Walking are physical, emotional, social, and spiritual. They include:
- improved bone density
- enhanced aerobic fitness
- lower blood pressure
- reduced risk of heart disease
- lower blood cholesterol
- increase in metabolism

- decreases in body fat (if you get to Fitness Zone)
- reduced stress
- improved sleep patterns and more restful sleep
- increased lung capacity
- revitalization

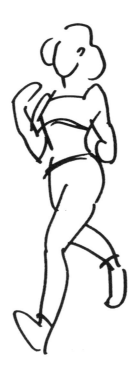

15-WEEK SMART WALKING PROGRAM

Use this 15-week program as a guide for the duration and frequency of exercise.

Week	1	2	3	4	5	6	7	8	9	10	11	12	13	14	15
Duration	10 min.	15 min.	15 min.	20 min.	20 min.	25 min.	25 min.	30 min.	30 min.	35 min.	35 min.	40 min.	40 min.	45 min.	45 min.
Times (per week)	3	3	4-5	3	4-5	3	4-5	3	4-5	3	4-5	3	4-5	3	4-5

After 15 weeks, walk 45 minutes 3-5 times a week to maintain fitness.

Meet Your Authors

Ronda Gates

Ronda Gates, M. S., C. L. C., is a health promotion educator whose company, LIFESTYLES by Ronda Gates, develops and delivers programs and products to support lifestyle change.

In 1978 Ronda exchanged the white coat she wore during her 17 year career as a hospital pharmacist for a pair of athletic shoes and never looked back. Her corporate fitness business precipitated graduate health studies, many prestigious awards and fellowships, and a professional career that reflects her effort to make sense out of the conflicting information, myths, and misconceptions about women's health. She is passionate about the mission of Speaking of Women's Health Foundation, which is one of the venues where she has an opportunity to lend her humorous perspective to serious topics related to women's health.

When Ronda is not "on the road" lecturing about the many aspects of making healthy lifestyle change, she is writing about it for publication in the press, magazines, and on the internet. She maintains her good bone health by teaching a daily dance fitness class and "re-creates" in her garden, on a bicycle, and hiking hills nationwide.

Ronda, the mother of two grown children, Rebecca and Caleb, lives in Lake Oswego, OR. You can learn more about her at the LIFESTYLES by Ronda Gates website: http://www.rondagates.com. She can be contacted at ronda@rondagates.com or 503-697-7572.

Beverly Whipple

Beverly Whipple, Ph.D., R. N., F.A.A.N., is Professor Emeritus, Rutgers University, Past-President of the American Association of Sex Educators, Counselors and Therapists and Vice-President, World Association for Sexology (2001–2005). She has devoted her professional life to conducting research, teaching, and speaking nationally and internationally about women's health issues and the sexuality and sensuality of women and couples.

You may know Beverly as the author of the international best-seller, The G Spot and Other Recent Discoveries about Human Sexuality. She is often the subject of feature articles in many of your favorite magazines. Beverly's ability to make sexual subjects that mystify women easy to understand is only one of her many skills. She enjoys using her understanding of complex research (her doctorate is in neurophysiology) to clarify health issues so women can learn about themselves and accept and enjoy the mysteries of womanhood. Her sense of humor and matter of fact, nonjudgmental style, have helped women world-wide to understand and deal with the complexities of life and their relationships.

Dr. Whipple has received numerous awards and fellowships for her research contributions to women's health. She lives in Medford, New Jersey with her husband, Jim. They have two grown children and four grandchildren. She can be contacted at bwhipple@recomnet.net or 609-953-1937.

For more about Beverly's perspective on sexual health visit www.sexualhealth.com.

Index

Profits from the sale of additional copies of *Smart Women, Strong Bones* will be donated to Speaking of Women's Health Foundation.

There are three convenient ways to order additional copies:
1. On the internet: http://www.rondagates.com
    • A secure site; use Smart Bargains icon
    or http//www.sexualhealth.com (the Sexual Health Network, Inc.)

2. By phone: 503-697-7572
    • Visa and MC accepted

3. By mail: C/O LIFESTYLES 4-Heart Press
            P.O. Box 974
            Lake Oswego, OR 97034

Each book costs $10.
Discounts for multiples of 10 or more.
Add $1.50 per book for regular shipping and handling.
Add $3.50 per book for priority mail and handling.

To ship your book(s) we need:
    Number of copies you wish to purchase
    Your Name
    Your Shipping Address
    Your Phone Number (in case there is a problem) or
    Your email address
    Your Visa or MC # and expiration date on the card
    The name on the credit card